Handbook of Sports Medicine and Science

Canoeing

Handbook of Sports Medicine and Science
Canoeing

EDITED BY

Don McKenzie, MD, PhD

Professor & Director
Division of Sport and Exercise Medicine
Faculty of Medicine & School of Kinesiology
The University of British Columbia, Vancouver, BC, Canada

Bo Berglund, MD, PhD

Associate Professor
Department of Medicine
Karolinska University Hospital, Solna, Sweden

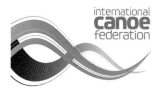

WILEY Blackwell

Registered Offices
John Wiley & Sons, Inc., 111 River Street, Hoboken, NJ 07030, USA
John Wiley & Sons Ltd, The Atrium, Southern Gate, Chichester, West Sussex, PO19 8SQ, UK

Editorial Office
9600 Garsington Road, Oxford, OX4 2DQ, UK

For details of our global editorial offices, customer services, and more information about Wiley products visit us at www.wiley.com.

Wiley also publishes its books in a variety of electronic formats and by print-on-demand. Some content that appears in standard print versions of this book may not be available in other formats.

Library of Congress Cataloging-in-Publication Data
Names: McKenzie, Don (Donald Chisholm), editor. | Berglund, Bo, 1948– editor.
Title: Canoeing / edited by Don McKenzie, Bo Berglund.
Description: Hoboken, NJ : Wiley-Blackwell, 2019. | Series: Handbook of sports
   medicine and science | Includes bibliographical references and index. |
Identifiers: LCCN 2018039259 (print) | LCCN 2018039946 (ebook) | ISBN 9781119097228
   (Adobe PDF) | ISBN 9781119097211 (ePub) | ISBN 9781119097204 (pbk.)
Subjects: | MESH: Water Sports–physiology | Water Sports–injuries | Water Sports–psychology
Classification: LCC GV783 (ebook) | LCC GV783 (print) | NLM QT 260 | DDC 797.122–dc23
LC record available at https://lccn.loc.gov/2018039259

Cover images: © International Olympic Committee
Cover design by Wiley

Set in 8.75/12pt ITC Stone Serif Std Medium by SPi Global, Pondicherry, India

Printed in Singapore by C.O.S. Printers Pte Ltd

10 9 8 7 6 5 4 3 2 1

Contents

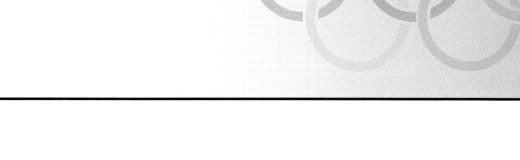

List of Contributors

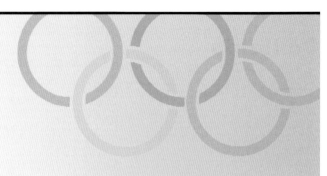

Bo Berglund, MD, PhD
Associate Professor, Department of Medicine,
Karolinska University Hospital, Solna, Sweden

Anna Bjerkefors, PhD, RPT
Senior Researcher, Lecturer, and Physiotherapist,
Swedish School of Sport and Health Sciences (GIH),
Laboratory of Biomechanics and Motor Control,
Stockholm, Sweden

Robert Boushel, DSc
Professor and Director, School of Kinesiology,
Faculties of Education and Medicine,
The University of British Columbia, Vancouver,
BC, Canada

Jose Calbet, MD, PhD
Department of Physical Education, University of Las
Palmas de Gran Canaria, Las Palmas de Gran Canaria,
Spain
Research Institute of Biomedical and Health Sciences
(IUIBS), University of Las Palmas de Gran Canaria, Las
Palmas de Gran Canaria, Spain

Sylvain Curinier, MS
Coach, National Canoe-Kayak Slalom, Fédération
Française de Canoë-Kayak (FFCK), Joinville-le-Pont,
France
Accompagnateur Coach, Diplomé de l'Executive
Master, INSEP, Paris, France
Practitioner, France PNL, Paris, France

Jozsef Dobos, MD
Department of Sport Surgery, National Institute of
Sports Medicine, Budapest, Hungary

John Edwards, BArch, BEd
Chair, ICF Paracanoe Committee, Mississippi Hills, ON,
Canada

Martin Hunter, MS, MA
Head Coach, Swedish Canoe Federation, Rosvalla, Sweden
Lecturer, School of Business, Örebro University, Örebro,
Sweden

Petra Lundström, PhLic
Department of Molecular Medicine and Surgery,
Karolinska Institute, Solna, Sweden

Don McKenzie, MD, PhD
Professor and Director, Division of Sport and Exercise
Medicine, Faculty of Medicine & School of Kinesiology,
The University of British Columbia, Vancouver,
BC, Canada

Kari-Jean McKenzie, MS, MD, FRCPC
Clinical Assistant Professor, Department of Medicine,
The University of British Columbia, Vancouver,
BC, Canada

Ian Mortimer, MA
Director of Development, Canoe Kayak Canada,
Ottawa, ON, Canada

Hans Rosdahl, PhD
Senior Lecturer, Swedish School of Sport and Health
Sciences (GIH), Stockholm, Sweden

Johanna Rosen, MSc
PhD Student, Sport Scientist, Swedish School of Sport
and Health Sciences (GIH), Laboratory of Biomechanics
and Motor Control, Stockholm, Sweden

A. William Sheel, PhD
Professor, School of Kinesiology, Faculty of Education,
The University of British Columbia, Vancouver,
BC, Canada

Jorunn Sundgot Borgen, PhD
Professor, Physical Activity and Health, Department of
Sports Medicine, Norwegian School of Sports Sciences,
Oslo, Norway

Olga Tarassova, MSc
Laboratory Engineer, Swedish School of Sport and
Health Sciences (GIH), Laboratory of Biomechanics and
Motor Control, Stockholm, Sweden

Barney Wainwright, PhD
Research Fellow, Leeds Beckett University, Carnegie
School of Sport, Leeds, UK

Penny Werthner, PhD
Professor and Dean, Faculty of Kinesiology, University
of Calgary, Calgary, AB, Canada

Foreword

As President of the International Canoe Federation (ICF), it is my pleasure to welcome you to this excellent canoe-focused publication that is part of the International Olympic Committee's Handbooks on Sports Medicine and Science series.

Canoeing has always had a strong image as a healthy sport combining the highest levels of athletic achievement with spectacular locations. Throughout history, the margin of success or failure within our sport has been slim, and nowhere is this more prevalent than at the very highest level, the Olympic Games.

Canoeing has a rich and long history within the Olympic movement, with canoe sprint being introduced in 1924 and then becoming a full medal sport by the Berlin 1936 Olympic Games.

Slalom's Olympic journey started later when it debuted at the 1972 Munich Olympic Games. It then returned when the Games moved to Barcelona in 1992 and has been one of the core sports ever since.

Both disciplines have benefited greatly from their connection to the world's largest sporting celebration, as have the other seven disciplines that operate under the banner of our International Federation.

However, long before any athlete wins the honor to represent their nation at the highest level, they will need to dedicate their life to their chosen sport,

each day honing their skills, refining their diet, and building their strength to compete with the world's best.

It is this part of an athlete's life that goes unseen – the hours, days, weeks, months, and years of preparation that make an Olympic champion. This is where this publication sits, taking world-leading medical research and distilling it into a practical application for everyone within our sport to benefit.

On behalf of the entire international canoe community, the ICF authorities, and our many canoeists, I would like to extend my gratitude and compliments to the authors. Their contribution and ability to gather and then articulate such a complex body of research in a manner suitable for all is an amazing achievement and will inevitably help to further enhance the global development of our sport.

I congratulate and thank all those involved with this outstanding publication.

With my compliments,

José Perurena
ICF President and IOC Member

Foreword

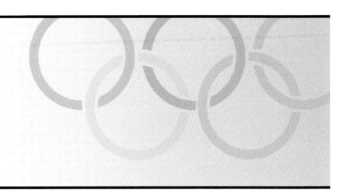

Canoeing and kayaking have been an important part of the Olympic competitions for 70 years, for both men and women. At the Rio 2016 Olympic Games, competitions were held for men and women in four events for slalom (3M–1W) and 12 for sprint (8M–4W); and six events for kayak were held in the 2016 Paralympic Games.

The aim of this Handbook is to present the latest research dealing with the medicine and science of canoeing, organized by topic area chapters and presented with practical applications. Dr. Don McKenzie (Canada) was selected as editor for the project, and he successfully assembled a team of contributing authors who provided authoritative coverage of all aspects of the medicine and science of canoe/kayak competition.

The Handbook will most certainly constitute an invaluable working tool and source of guidance for medical doctors, related health personnel, and coaches who work with the athletes who participate at the international, national, and regional levels of competition. By joining the International Olympic Committee (IOC) Medical and Scientific Commission's Handbooks of Sports Medicine and Science series, this Handbook will serve as an important source of sports medicine and sports science information for many years to come.

Thomas Bach
IOC President

Preface

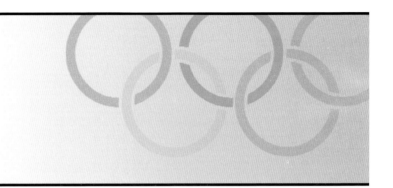

Few activities connect you to the environment like canoeing. As a sport, competitive canoe and kayak racing is unique, given the range of craft and water conditions. The International Canoe Federation is the governing body and provides leadership in nine disciplines. ParaCanoe, sprint, and slalom are well known due to their inclusion in the Olympic program. In these events, success is decided by objective measurement of time to complete a distance or course. The physical and mental preparation to compete is extreme, and these athletes challenge the limits of human performance. Control and integration of many factors are necessary to reach the podium.

The other disciplines are no less demanding. Marathon events require technical skill, tactics, and endurance over many kilometers. Freestyle competition involves acrobatics performed in whitewater on stationary river features. Points are given for spins, turns, and flips accumulated in a 60-second routine. Wild water competition represents the purity of effort, while racing downriver in class 2 to 4 whitewater. In Canoe ocean racing, competitors race in surfskis, sea kayaks, and single and six-person outriggers exposed to the wind and waves of the open ocean. There is a distinctive field of play and competition between teams in

Canoe polo. Teams of five-paddlers strive to score a ball into a net suspended above the water at each end of the pitch. Dragon boat has links to the cultural and traditional components of Canoeing. Originating in China more than 2000 years ago, current racing involves teams of 10 or 20 paddlers competing over distances from 200 to 2000 m.

This Handbook represents the efforts of experts in all areas of medicine and science applied to Canoeing. It provides general information on the history and development of Canoeing as well as specific chapters with concise, but detailed, information on sport science and the clinical aspects of Canoe sport. It is hoped that this Handbook will provide useful information to the athlete, coach, and support personnel as well as the reader interested in competitive and recreational canoeing.

It is a privilege to be included in the IOC series of Handbooks of Sports Medicine and Science. On behalf of the authors, we are indebted to Dr. Skip Knuttgen, paddler, scientist, and friend, who has guided us through the muddy waters of creating this Handbook. His expertise speaks for itself, and we owe him our gratitude.

Don McKenzie
2018

Chapter 1
Introduction

Ian Mortimer[1] and Don McKenzie[2]

[1]Canoe Kayak Canada, Ottawa, ON, Canada

[2]Division of Sport and Exercise Medicine, The University of British Columbia, Vancouver, BC, Canada

Introduction

Bodies of water, great and small, are a formative feature of the human experience on our blue planet. At every corner of the earth, people have been drawn to live near these sources of life. This connection between humankind and the seas, oceans, and rivers that we call home is reflected in a seemingly universal reaction to not just live by and immerse ourselves in water, but also find a way to float on its surface.

Simple watercraft, the technological step beyond swimming, are a fixture in the history of the human experience. Dugout canoes, reed rafts, framed boats covered with bark or animal skins, and simple wood-plank boats exist in as many varied forms as the unique bodies of water they float on and the myriad tasks they have been built to accomplish. Be it carrying a passenger to a far shore, collecting fish on a flowing stream, navigating the swell of the ocean, or traveling great distances on a flowing river, simple craft of simple means have existed for millennia in cultures around the world. These simplest of boats all share a core concept: a buoyant craft, a paddler or group of paddlers, and their paddles, allowing people to travel where feet, wheels, or hooves will not carry them. There is a fundamental joy in conquering our natural inability to move across the waters'

surface, a joy that never gets old. Paddlers of these craft the world over connect in this wonder, and most cannot help but smile at the sight of any type of paddled craft drifting into shore at sunset, shooting down a rapid in flood, or charging through an ocean swell.

The draw of the simplicity and universality of the paddle, paddler, and boat is an important part of the story of canoeing as a sport. However, the more specific story of competitive canoeing and kayaking traces its history through the canoe's part in the foundational myth of modern North America. Understanding the story of canoeing necessitates an understanding of the canoe itself as part of the protracted, and fraught, process of cultural contact between North American indigenous people and the European settler society. The names *canoe* and *kayak* themselves reflect this Euro-centric mindset of "discovery" of these indigenous craft and their peoples, with the words we have today emerging through the process of European languages wrestling the indigenous names into European vernacular. Christopher Columbus is credited with first encountering the Haitian word *canaoua* as a name for the dugout-type canoes of the island of Hispaniola, and bringing the term into Spanish as *canoa*, which came to the English as *canoe*, while the Greenlandic Inuit word for "small boats of skins," *qayaq*, returned to Europe with the Danes as *kajak*, which became *kayak*.

From the earliest stages of cultural contact, the unique adaptation of indigenous paddle-driven craft to perform in the waters of North America was quickly obvious to those who were arriving from across the ocean. This was especially apparent on the inland waterways of the continent, where the major rivers, now known as the St. Lawrence, Ottawa, Hudson, Ohio, Mississippi, and Missouri, and their hundreds of smaller tributaries served as highways of canoe travel. It became clear to the European colonizers, explorers, and traders that adopting the light, repairable, and maneuverable canoes they learned to build and paddle from the Mi'kmaq, Wendat, Haudenosaunee, and others was the only efficient way to travel the expanses of the North American landmass.

The canoe became a critical feature in the life of any European looking to travel beyond the salty waters of their continent's shore, and indeed was a foundation in the process of exploration, expansion, and eventual domination of the North American landmass by European settlers. Canoes took Lewis and Clarke across the American continent and carried David Thompson on his lifelong mission to map what is now the Canadian West. Meanwhile, for over 200 years the fur trade of beaver pelts, which was the backbone of the economy of British North America, operated using a variety of sizes of canoes and a vast network of routes. The Hudson's Bay Company, deeded by the British Crown to carry out this trade, and its eventual rival the North-West Company, used canoes to carry information, supplies, and furs across thousands of kilometers of rivers and lakes from present-day Montreal to the Rocky Mountains. For two centuries ending in the mid-1800s, being a professional paddler, or *voyageur*, was a viable career in New France and British North America for European, Aboriginal, and Métis men and women alike (Figure 1.1).

With this history and the mythology around it, the canoe holds heavy significance as a cultural marker for North America. The silhouette of the classic canoe, with its upturned stern and bow, is an iconic image associated with wilderness, exploration, and indigenous people. It is important to think critically about this significance and the cultural

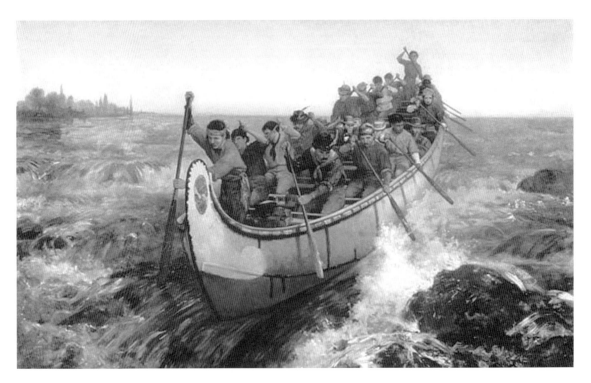

Figure 1.1 A *canot du maître*, the large canoes used in the North American fur trade to travel major river routes.

place that the canoe holds not just for North America generally, but for Aboriginal peoples specifically. The mythology of the canoe can be a point of friction in the relationship between settler society and indigenous North American culture. There is no doubt that a debt of gratitude must be given for the gift of these ingenious North American boats to the world, and respect for the beauty reflected in their varied designs, refined for the landscape they were developed in through the ages.

By the late 1800s, the fur trade in North America was well past its prime. Rail lines stretched across the continent, and the highways of water were supplanted once and for all by these ribbons of steel. Along with Europe, North America was changing. The industrial revolution had fundamentally altered the economies on both sides of the Atlantic, and a new lifestyle awaited those who emerged through these changes as the middle class developed. With population shifts to cities, a wider distribution of wealth, more young people seeking education, and fewer hours needed for manual labor, the widespread concept of leisure time and recreation took off. Most major traditional sports we recognize today were born during this era. For the team sport and rule-minded athlete, baseball and football developed in North America while soccer (football) was rapidly gaining popularity in Europe. For those craving speed and modernity, there was the new sport of cycling. There was rowing, a mainstay at collegiate levels, and certainly the more technologically advanced of the water sports. Yet for those who sought to connect with water, but in a simpler craft, there was the sport of canoeing.

In America, where the mythology of the rugged paddlers of the era of exploration and the fur trade was strong, canoeing offered a connection to a nostalgic past. The living experience in cities like New York, Montreal, Ottawa, and Washington less and less resembled this conception of a wild and heroic past linked to generations gone by. Weekend trips to a lake or river to go canoeing became a popular chance to bridge the gap with the imagined past, feel authentically rugged, and enjoy the natural landscape increasingly distant from city life. Some sought out quiet lakes for sunset cruises, while others searched for the whirling rapids of the springtime melt. New canoes based on those of the fur trade and traditional Aboriginal designs, but updated for speed, whitewater, or comfort, were created using new materials and techniques, yet the core simplicity of boat, paddle, and paddler remained. For Europeans, canoeing was an activity that got them out of the city to float on country rivers, and the ponds of city parks. But it was also a chance to experience a piece of an "authentic" North American–style adventure, to feel a connection to the stories of the wilds of the continent across the ocean, and to re-create that imagined, idealized simple life of the Aboriginal peoples that they would read about in adventure novels. The style of boats being produced for purely recreational purposes in North America were brought to European waters, and they proved popular with the newly conceived figure of the weekend warrior who would flee the city on precious days off for some country air and a vigorous paddle.

On both sides of the ocean canoe clubs sprang up, founded by canoeing enthusiasts. These clubs were more than just boathouses in which to store canoes. By offering members access to boats, they provided the opportunity for a wider public to experience the sport, and out of this camaraderie the clubs became social hubs for their members during the summer months (Figures 1.2 and 1.3). These early clubs would be instrumental in the genesis of canoe racing we know today. In England, the first formal club was the Royal Canoe Club on the Thames, founded in 1866. It was home to the formative pioneer of canoe design, touring, and competition, John "Rob Roy" MacGregor. The first club in the United States, the New York Canoe Club, followed in 1870, and in Canada the earliest canoe club was built in this same period at the entrance to the Lachine Canal on the Island of Montreal. Soon, other clubs sprung up both in England and in Eastern North America, and before long the competitive spirit of these clubs' members, and the pride in their home clubs' colors, began to take effect. Races were organized, and over time competitive rivalries evolved. By the turn of the twentieth century, these clubs and early races had sparked formal national associations that went on to publish rule books, designate officials, and hold annual regattas. The sport of canoe and kayak racing as we know it today at the international level was born (Figure 1.4).

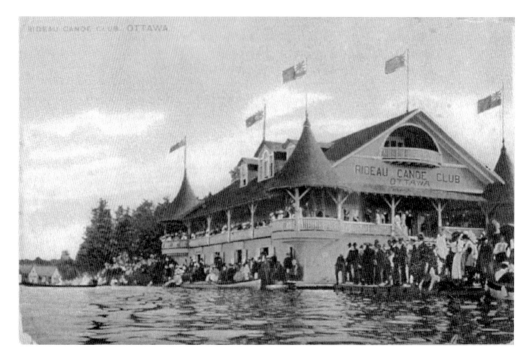

Figure 1.2 The packed docks and deck of the Rideau Canoe Club on Regatta Day 1906 illustrate the popularity of canoe clubs as social as well as sporting hubs at the turn of the twentieth century.

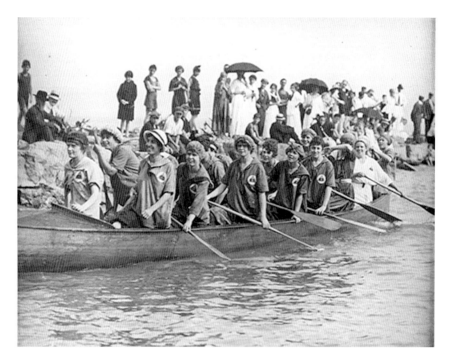

Figure 1.3 Although dominated by men, the earliest stages of organized, competitive canoe racing included women. War canoe racing in Canada, circa 1909.

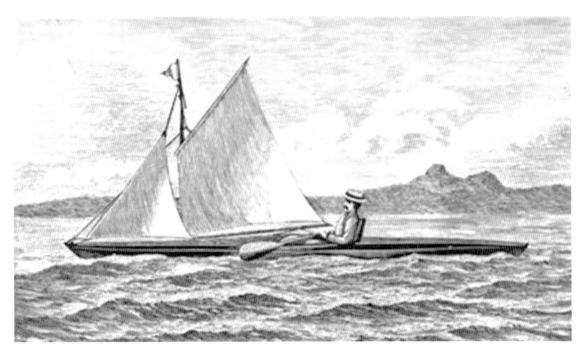

Figure 1.4 John MacGregor, founder of the British Royal Canoe Club, in the *Rob Roy*.

Internationalia Represantantskapet for Kanotidrott (IRK)

In the early 1900s, with the rapid expansion of canoe clubs and the increasing popularity of the activity, there was a need for structure, not just to organize international competitions but also to advise the public on items such as touring, sightseeing, international signs for maps, safety, and so on. In January 1924, representatives from four National Federations (Austria, Denmark, Germany, and Sweden) met in Copenhagen at what was the First Congress. They formed the IRK and adopted statutes that established the purpose and vision of this organization:

- To form links amongst National Federations and organize international competitions in canoeing and sailing.
- International categories were established for competition paddling canoes (single-seat kayak: maximum length 5.20 m, maximum width 0.51 m) and sailing canoes. Dimensions of the Canadian canoe were deferred until the American Canoe Association could be consulted.
- The international paddling races were from 1500 to 10 000 m, and the sailing competition was on a triangular course of a minimum of 10 km, with one side facing the wind.
- To promote touring, including sightseeing, accommodation, and maps.

In the early years of the IRK, the focus was on providing leadership to the sport in terms of equipment like tandem kayaks and folding boats, and promotion of activities such as international canoe camping tours. Canoe clubs flourished and became gathering places for canoeing as well as social activities.

Competitive canoeing developed with each International Canoe Federation (ICF) Congress. Canoe slalom was established in 1931 on Lake Hallwyl in Switzerland by Max Vogt, and the first wild water slalom followed in 1933 on the Arr River. The first World Championships were in Geneva in 1949. Gradually, as the different disciplines evolved and established a competitive presence with individual regattas, the ICF recognized each one at a Congress. Technical committees were established, rules published, championships announced, and the world of canoe sport evolved, all under the guidance of the ICF.

The initial Flatwater Championships took place in Vaxholm, in the Sweden archipelago, in 1938. Athletes competed on the ocean, and accommodation was nearby in tents (Figures 1.5–1.7).

Canoe sailing dates to the very early days of the nineteenth century with John McGregor in the United Kingdom. The first ICF World Championship was in 1961 and is held every three years. Long-distance paddling has an extensive history, and both marathon and wildwater canoeing grew from these distance races. Classic wildwater canoeing had its first World Championship in 1959; Marathon

was recognized as an official discipline by the ICF in 1984, and World Championships for it were introduced at that time. Canoe polo became popular in the mid-twentieth century, and the ICF published the rules for this sport in 1986; the first World Championship took place in 1994. Dragon Boat was added to the list of sanctioned disciplines in 2004 and has World Championships each year. The ICF recognized Freestyle as an official discipline in 2006, and the first canoe freestyle World Championship was held in 2007. Ocean racing was a natural extension of marathon and involves long-distance surf ski and Va'a competitions. Ocean Racing is the newest discipline in the ICF, bringing the current number to 10.

In 1964, at the Congress in Tokyo, a Sport Medicine Committee was established, and two years later doping controls were initiated. This was the second International Federation to realize the importance of medicine in sport and to recognize the potential problem of drugs in sport. Since that time, the ICF has had a zero-tolerance policy toward doping in sport and has mandatory educational programs prior to competition.

The growth of the ICF was slow until the 1990s, when development programs were funded to introduce the sport throughout the world. The initial Congress had 4 National Federations, and even at the 50th Anniversary of the ICF in 1974, only 31 Federations attended the Congress. However, the growth in the last 30 years has been rapid, and, at this time, 167 National Federations in 5 continents hold membership in the ICF.

Canoeing as an Olympic sport

In the year that the IRK was founded, there were demonstration races in kayak and canoe at the eighth Olympic Games in Paris. The International Olympic Committee's (IOC) Organizing Committee contacted the Canadian Olympic Committee, who sent competitors from the Canadian Canoe Association and the Washington Canoe Club to participate in six events. Races in singles, doubles, and fours, in both canoe and kayak, were incorporated into the Olympic Rowing regatta on July 13

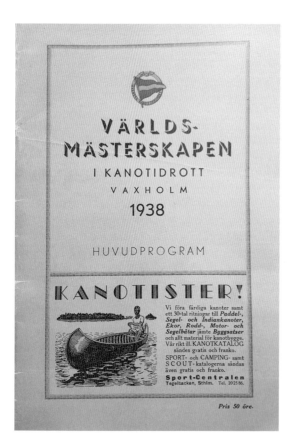

Figure 1.5 Announcement of the first ICF Flatwater Championship in Sweden, 1938.

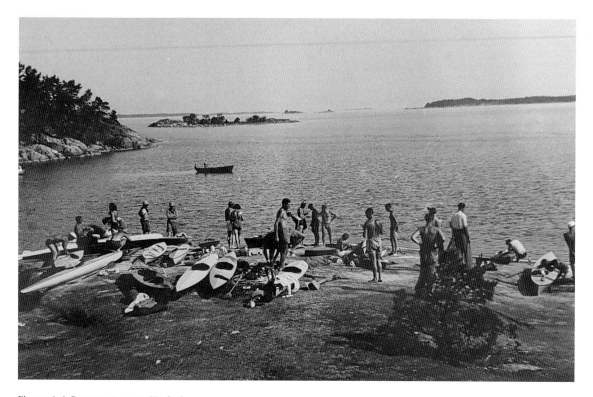

Figure 1.6 Regatta site near Vaxholm.

and 15, 1924. Although this would seem to indicate that canoeing would be admitted to the Olympic program, such was not the case. Applications to the IOC were rejected for the 1928 and 1932 Games, largely because of the small number of National Federations. Dr. Max Eckert, the President of the German Canoe Federation, was elected President of the IRK at the 1932 Congress in Vienna. At that meeting, all efforts were directed toward a strategy that would lead to the admission of canoeing to the 1936 Games in Berlin. A decision was made to hold the first European Championship in Prague in 1933 to place canoeing on the international stage; nine nations participated. Races were held for men over 10000 and 1000 m in kayak singles, folding singles, and folding pairs, and Canadian canoe singles and pairs. For women, there was one kayak singles race over 600 m. It would be a long, upstream battle for gender equity in canoe sport.

All National Federations that were part of the IRK were encouraged to apply to the IOC, through their own National Olympic Committee, for inclusion of canoeing in the Berlin Games. However, the IOC again rejected the application in 1933, and the Fédération Internationale des Sociétés d'Aviron (FISA, the international rowing federation) President was instrumental in this decision. Representing the opinion of many rowing federations, he was concerned that canoeists would compromise the freedom of lakes and waterways with the new influx of small craft. His argument against inclusion in the Olympics was that canoe racing was too young and not a competitive sport, nor was it prepared for such a great event. Not unexpectedly, the IRK responded with strong arguments to the contrary and launched an appeal to the IOC that was put on the agenda of the next IOC Congress in 1934. Finally, on May 16, 1934, the IOC agreed to accept the application from the IRK under the official Olympic name "Federation Internationale de Canoe" (FIC). There would be nine canoeing events in the 1936 Games in Berlin, but no women's race (Figures 1.8 and 1.9).

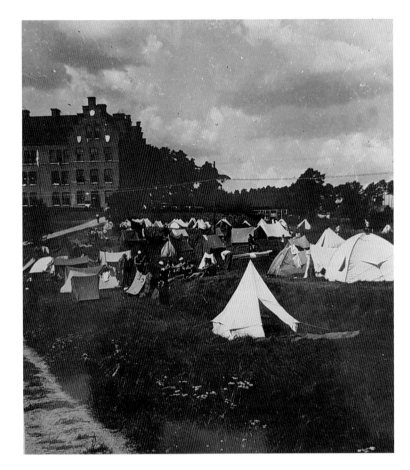

Figure 1.7 Tent accommodation near the regatta venue.

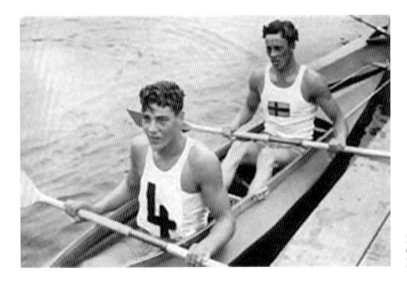

Figure 1.8 Competitors in the 1936 Olympic Games. This is a 10000 m kayak folding-boat double event.

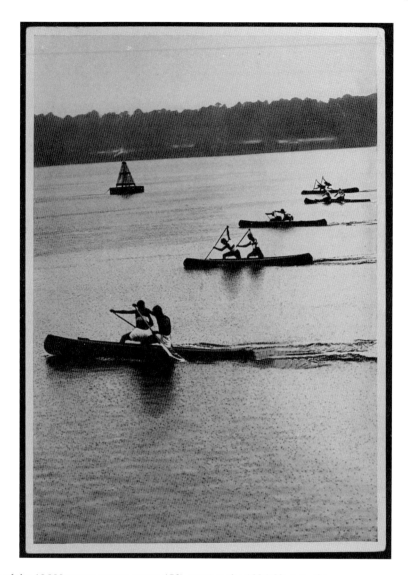

Figure 1.9 Start of the 10 000 m two-person canoe (C2) event at the 1936 Olympic Games.

Table 1.1 Slalom Olympic program.

	1972	...	1996	2000	2004	2008	2012	2016	2020
C1 M	X		X	X	X	X	X	X	X
C2 M	X		X	X	X	X	X	X	
K1 M	X		X	X	X	X	X	X	X
K1 W	X		X	X	X	X	X	X	X
C1 W									X
Number of events	4		4	4	4	4	4	4	4

1, One-person; 2, two-person; C, canoe; K, kayak; M, men; W, women.

Table 1.2 Sprint Olympic program.

	1936	1948	1952	1956	1960	1964	1968	1972	1976	1980	1984	1988	1992	1996	2000	2004	2008	2012	2016	2020
Sprint Olympic program: men																				
K1 200m																		X	X	X
K2 200m																		X	X	
K1 500m									X	X	X	X	X	X	X	X	X			
K2 500m									X	X	X	X	X	X	X	X	X			
K1 1000m	X	X	X	X	X	X	X	X	X	X	X	X	X	X	X	X	X	X	X	X
K2 1000m	X	X	X	X	X	X	X	X	X	X	X	X	X	X	X	X	X	X	X	X
K1 10000m	X	X	X	X																
K1 4×500m relay					X															
K4 1000m						X	X	X	X	X	X	X	X	X	X	X	X	X	X	
K4 500m																				X
K1 folding 10000m	X																			
K2 folding 10000m	X																			
C1 200m																		X	X	
C1 500m									X	X	X	X	X	X	X	X	X			
C2 500m									X	X	X	X	X	X	X	X	X			
C1 1000m	X	X	X	X	X	X	X	X	X	X	X	X	X	X	X	X	X	X	X	X
C2 1000m	X	X	X	X	X	X	X	X	X	X	X	X	X	X	X	X	X	X	X	X
C1 10000m		X	X	X																
C2 10000m	X	X	X	X																
Number of events	8	7	7	7	5	5	5	5	9	9	9	9	9	9	9	9	9	8	8	6
Sprint Olympic program: women																				
K1 200m																		X	X	X
K1 500m		X	X	X	X	X	X	X	X	X	X	X	X	X	X	X	X	X	X	X
K2 500m					X	X	X	X	X	X	X	X	X	X	X	X	X	X	X	X
K4 500m											X	X	X	X	X	X	X	X	X	X
C1 200m																				X
C2 500m																				X
Number of events		1	1	1	2	2	2	2	2	2	3	3	3	3	3	3	3	4	4	6

1, One-person; 2, two-person; C, canoe; K, kayak; M, men; W, women.

Table 1.3 Past and present ICF Presidents.

1924–1925	Franz Reinecke	GER
1925–1928	Paul Wulff	DEN
1928–1932	Franz Reinecke	GER
1932–1945	Max W. Eckert	GER
1946–1949	Jonas Asschier	SWE
1950–1954	Harald Jespersen	DEN
1954–1960	Karel Popel	TCH
1960–1981	Charles de Coquereaumont	FRA
1981–1998	Sergio Orsi	ITA
1998–2008	Ulrich Feldhoff	GER
2008–	Jose Perureno Lopez	ESP

After these Games, there was a large gap in competitive canoe sport, largely because of the war. The next Olympic Games were in 1948 and included a one-person kayak (K1) 500 m race for women. In 1960 a two-person kayak (K2) 500 m event was added, and in 1984 the four-person kayak (K4) 500 m race was added to the Olympic program in Los Angeles. The Olympic program remained unchanged until 2012, when all four men's 500 m races were eliminated and replaced by K1, K2, and one-person canoe (C1) 200 m men's events, and a women's K1 200 m event. This schedule was maintained for the 2016 Games in Rio; however, further changes are planned for the 2020 Olympic Games in Tokyo. This will result in an equal number of races for women and men in both slalom and sprint competitions (Tables 1.1 and 1.2), including women's canoe.

The ICF has been fortunate to have capable leadership (Table 1.3). This has been necessary and instrumental in guiding the sport through periods of rapid growth and diversification. As canoeing remains one of the fastest growing activities in the world, guidance and governance remain high priorities.

In the twenty-first century, our view of the world of canoeing is constantly expanding. There are infinite varieties of paddling with their own rich stories and histories, all shaped by their own geographic region, type of water, and cultural and historical perspectives. Yet what unites all types of canoeing is that simple core concept of boat, paddler, and paddle. This shared simplicity of paddling a watercraft, and the unique feeling and wonder at pushing off from shore and paddling across the waters, is continually being reinforced.

Bibliography

Canoeing and Olympism. (1985) [Retrospective study, 1924–1985]. In: *Olympic encyclopedia: canoe: supplement to the Olympic Review*. Olympic Rev, 1985 Nov–Dec (Suppl.):1–56.

International Canoe Federation. www.canoeicf.com

Vesper, H.E. (1984). *Canoeing: 50 years of the International Canoe Federation*. Florence: International Canoe Federation.

Chapter 2
Biomechanics and equipment (sprint and slalom): a review of scientifically confirmed information

Barney Wainwright
Leeds Beckett University, Carnegie School of Sport, Leeds, UK

CANOE SPRINT

Equipment

The choice of equipment that an athlete makes for sprint racing is determined by the aim of completing the race distance in as little time as possible. In terms of a boat choice, this would be one that minimizes drag yet provides a sufficiently stable platform that enables the athlete to reliably create frequent, forceful, and effective paddle strokes. The paddle should be of a size (length and blade area) and shape that suits the athletes' individual anthropometric and muscle characteristics, as well as their paddling style. It goes without saying that the equipment chosen must conform to the International Canoe Federation's (ICF) racing rules (see http://www.canoeicf.com/icf/AboutICF/Rules-and-Statutes.html).

Historical changes in equipment and performance times

The development and evolution of equipment have not always been driven by scientific advances, with most developments occurring through intuition and trial and error by small groups of committed innovators, with science only retrospectively proving a justification for the designs. Many of the advances in equipment were only made possible as improved manufacturing techniques and materials, such as fiberglass and carbon fiber, became available. As a result, the choice of equipment available to athletes has changed over the years (Table 2.1). Although it is obvious that the developments in equipment have, in general, led to improved racing times, the relationship between the two is not always apparent (see the historical race times charts in Figures 2.4–2.6).

Boats

In recent years, the most significant change came about in late 1998, when the boat manufacturer Plastex stretched the limits of the rules by raising the deck in the area of minimum width. This design change allowed the boat to conform to the minimum width rules, and effectively created a narrower waterline width. In November 2000, the ICF removed the minimum width rule from the rules, which meant that the "peaked decks" could be removed, and the boats regained their more traditional look. The additional benefit has been for smaller athletes who have been able to use boats with smaller cross-sectional areas, thus becoming more competitive. The resulting reduction in the height of the hull sides considerably eased steering

Canoeing, First Edition. Edited by Don McKenzie and Bo Berglund.
© 2019 International Olympic Committee. Published 2019 by John Wiley & Sons Ltd.

Table 2.1 The major events in the development of equipment in canoe sprint (Figures 2.1–2.3).

1936: Paris	1000 m events in rigid boats.
1948: London	Boats used were very high volume – a style that remained in use until the late 1950s.
1952: Helsinki	C1 beam reduced to 0.75 m. V-form hulls introduced.
1956: Melbourne	Concave decklines appeared in K1s, allowing paddles to get closer to the center line.
1960: Rome	Square-ended blades started to be replaced by asymmetric-shaped blades. Struer introduced the "Fighter" K1, which had an underwater form similar to that of contemporary boats.
1964: Tokyo	C2 length changed to 6.5 m, and width to 0.75 m. No concave rule introduced, so diamond-shaped kayaks evolved as a result. The boat design remained fairly stable until 2000.
1968: Mexico City	First time a purpose-built regatta course was used.
1972: Munich	Fiberglass boats started to appear. Struer introduced the Delta-shaped Lancer in 1969.
1980: Moscow	Boat surface control was introduced.
1984: Los Angeles	Fiberglass paddles started to be the predominant choice of material for kayaks.
1988: Seoul	NZ speed pods attempted to be used, but were not allowed. Van Dusen Eagle boats introduced. Wing paddles adopted by most top-level paddlers.
1996: Atlanta	Last time kayak races were won in wooden boats. K1 1000 m (Holmann), K1 500 m (Rossi). Composite manufacture allowed more ergonomic shapes to be used, such as scooped-out foredecks to allow the blade to get closer to the center line.
2000: Sydney	Boats with raised decks to circumnavigate the minimum width rule dominated. Carbon fiber–based composite boats widespread. The C1 Delta was replaced by newer designs.
2004: Athens	The minimum width rule was abolished in late 2000, allowing more traditional deck shapes to be reintroduced.
2015	Nelo released the Cinco, an inverted bow design – the most radical design change since 2000. C1 weight restriction decreased to 14 kg from 16 kg.

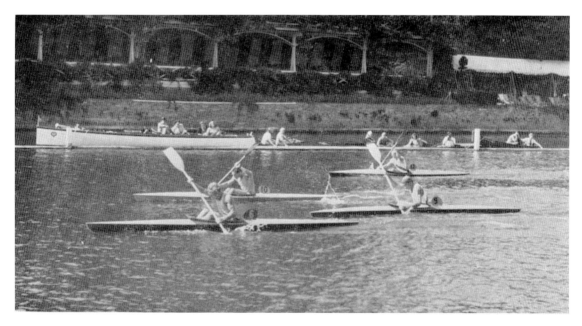

Figure 2.1 Gert Fredriksson (no. 6) making the amazing spurt that gave him victory in the men's K1 1000 m event at the 1948 Olympics at Henley, UK. *Source*: Courtesy of the ICF.

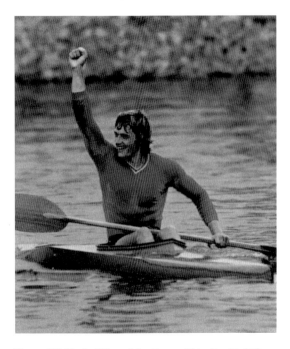

Figure 2.2 Vasile Diba celebrating gold in the K1 500 m at the Montreal Olympics in 1976. He paddles a wooden Lancer-type boat (delta shape) with wooden paddles. *Source*: Courtesy of the ICF.

mum beam has been reduced (from approximately 1999 onward), the performance times have remained fairly stable in each of the categories. Since then, changes in hull design have been subtle, with designers experimenting with changes in the rocker, distribution of prismatic volume, and cross-sectional shape to maximize the efficiency of the crew by reducing boat movement as much as possible. Following the use of computational flow dynamics (CFD) modeling and improved manufacturing techniques in recent years, opportunities for significant reductions in drag are generally considered to be limited until a rule change permits more extreme deviations from the current designs. One recent development by Nelo, the Cinco, introduced early in 2015, has been the use of an "inverted bow" (Figure 2.7), which is purported to reduce drag by allowing the bow wave to ride high up onto the sides of the kayak, reducing wave drag and pitching. It is yet to be seen whether this design improves performance, as essentially while wave drag may be reduced, friction drag due to an increased whetted area is increased. It may well be that the magnitude of any advantages is lost in less than perfect conditions.

The addition of the 200 m racing distance to the Olympic program, which was first contested in 2012, has led to some subtle design changes from various boat manufacturers. There has, however, been an increased emphasis on ensuring that

issues in crosswinds for canoes in particular, and reduced the stress levels of those responsible for loading boats onto trailers at the end of races! Figures 2.4–2.6 show that since the effective mini-

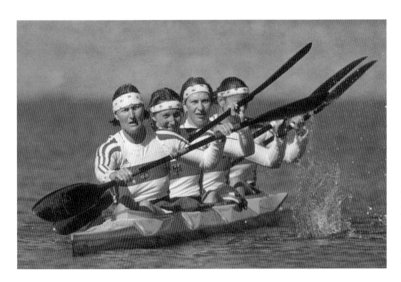

Figure 2.3 Fischer, Mucke, Wagner, and Schuck (representing Germany) won gold in the WK4 500 m event at the 2000 Sydney Olympics. Note the use of a "raised-deck" toward the stern of the boat to meet the minimum width requirements in place at the time. *Source*: Courtesy of the IOC.

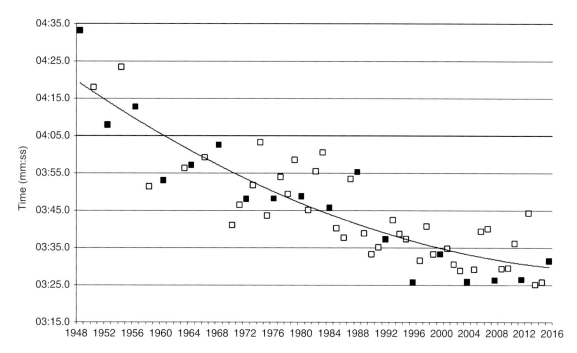

Figure 2.4 Men's K1 1000 m winning race times at Olympics (filled markers) and World Championships (open markers). In 1948, the races were held against the flow of the River Thames, and the effect of altitude at the Mexico City Olympics in 1968 caused relatively slower times.

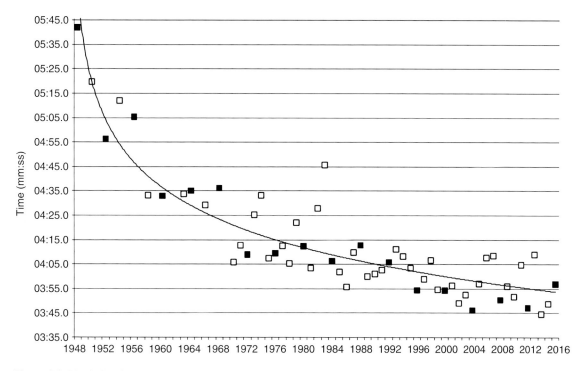

Figure 2.5 Men's C1 1000 m winning race times at Olympics (filled markers) and World Championships (open markers) from 1948 to 2015. In 1948, the races were held against the flow of the River Thames, and the effect of altitude at the Mexico City Olympics in 1968 caused relatively slower times.

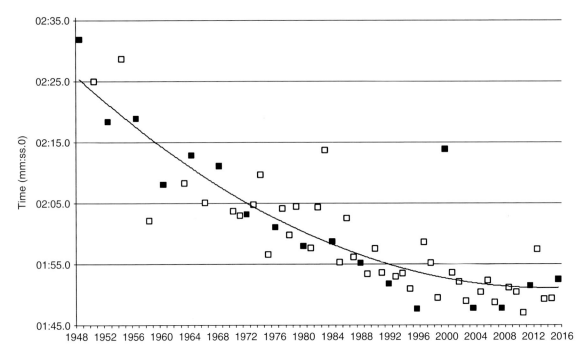

Figure 2.6 Women's K1 500 m winning race times at Olympics (filled markers) and World Championships (open markers) from 1948 to 2015. There was a strong headwind in this event at the Sydney Olympics, which had a large influence on the winning time.

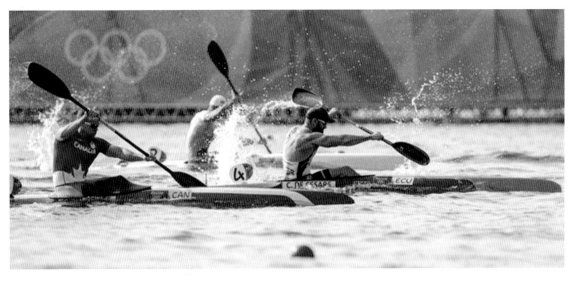

Figure 2.7 The Nelo Cinco with the "inverted bow" in use in the men's kayak 200 m at the Rio Olympics. *Source:* Balint Vekassy, © ICF.

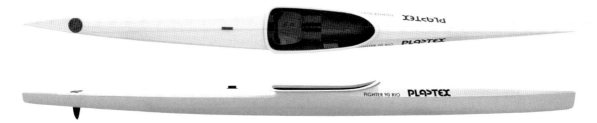

Figure 2.8 Contemporary racing kayak single (K1). *Source*: Courtesy of the ICF.

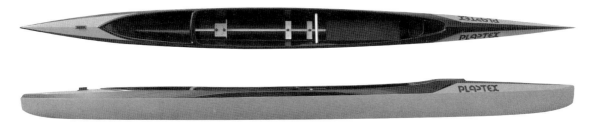

Figure 2.9 Contemporary racing canoe single (C1). *Source*: Courtesy of the ICF.

the boat's trim, determined by the position of the center of mass relative to the length of the boat, is correct for the individual athlete and the speed at which they are traveling. It has been suggested that the increased boat speed found in 200 m races causes the rear section of the boat to be sucked downward to a great extent, causing a larger increase in drag than would be expected if the boat was to maintain its normal profile (Figures 2.8 and 2.9).

Paddles

Since the first formal competitions in the early twentieth century, the small changes in paddle design are unlikely to have had a significant effect on performance. Paddles were essentially flat and made of wood, but the smaller stepwise reductions in weight and shape will have made small contributions to improvements in performance. As fiberglass paddles were introduced, their benefits were not immediately apparent, as often the early construction methods and materials offered no clear advantage. In 1986, the Swedish "wing" paddle was produced, which was the first major advance-

ment in improving the propulsive efficiency. This new paddle, which required a change in paddling technique, soon gained acceptance and was used by the majority of competitors at the Seoul Olympics in 1988. The racing paddles used now are essentially derivations of this original design. Further developments have occurred, with paddles now made exclusively of carbon fiber with a number of options for size and shape. When considering the race times (Figures 2.4–2.6), the performance improvements that may have occurred as a direct result of the introduction of the wing paddle are not obvious. This is even more apparent when compared with the decrease in performance times in the canoe class during the same period, when they had no similar evolution in paddle design. Although there has been little research comparing the standard flat asymmetric paddle with a wing-type paddle, what little research there has been has found an improvement in propulsive efficiency. Jackson et al. (1992) carried out a number of tests and calculated that the modern "wing-style" blade had an efficiency of 89% versus 75% for a standard "flat" blade. Given the complexities of paddle propulsion along with the different styles of technique and individual differences in power and body size, obtaining the optimal benefit from paddles is not straightforward. Canoe paddles have remained relatively unchanged for many years. Those used are relatively "flat," but are now made of carbon instead of wood, although even now some high-level athletes use paddles with wooden blades. Although canoe blades are generally rectangular in shape with little spoon, recently many high-level athletes have started to prefer the wider and more square-shaped models that are available, which are reported to load the start of the stroke or "catch."

Biomechanics

The paddling style that is adopted by an individual is determined by the technique required for that event (e.g. single canoe [C1] sprint 1000 m); the individual's own characteristics in terms of body dimensions, strength characteristics, flexibility, and stability; as well as any constraints created by the equipment that is being used. The generalized technique for that particular event has evolved to be as effective as possible while being governed by the underlying biomechanics. So, we can see that the style, technique, and biomechanics are very related, and by understanding the biomechanics that governs an event, the rationale for a particular technique and individual style can be understood and the optimization of a paddler can begin from a coaching perspective. The mechanical principles that underpin a particular movement are often not well understood, and sometimes ignored, with direct technique interventions taking place. This has often led coaches to pay a lot of attention to minor details of the stroke that actually have little effect on boat speed. If a better grasp of the key mechanical factors were had, a coach and athlete could spend their time and energy more effectively. Having said that, there is very little canoeing- or kayaking-specific mechanical information available for coaches or science and medicine practitioners, so it is not surprising that coaches and athletes find it difficult to prioritize or clearly identify what aspects of their technique they should be aiming to change. The aim of this section is to describe the key biomechanical factors that underpin canoeing and kayaking that will help athlete, coaches, and practitioners understand the basis of the environment in which they operate.

Fluid mechanics

The water and air provide resistive forces to movement. In the case of canoe sprint, the resistance is, in most circumstances, acting straight against the direction of travel. The factors that determine drag in canoe sprint have been identified by Jackson (1995) and are displayed in Figure 2.10. While some of these factors are relatively fixed, such as waterline length, some can be altered. For example, the paddler may be able to lose body weight that would reduce the volumetric displacement of the hull, reducing friction drag and hull drag. The result would be a faster traveling velocity as long as all other inputs remained the same. In the same manner, the reduction in the minimum mass from 16 to 14 kg in the C1 class should lead to very slightly faster racing times. Changes in environmental conditions such as water temperature (which affects water density), air temperature (which affects air density), and wind speed and direction all account for a majority of the differences in race times that occur between regattas. World record times are generally recorded when the environmental conditions are such that drag is low. Obviously, all types of drag (friction, wave, and aerodynamic) will increase as the boat travels at faster speeds.

Table 2.2 shows some values for the main components of drag for the men's and women's kayak classes given typical inputs for boat speed and crew mass. These were calculated by Jackson (1995), who used standardized equations and the specific class dimensions and inputs. Although they are based upon a modeling procedure, the results do allow us to understand the differences in drag that can occur due to different speeds and crew masses, as well as the differences between classes. Recently, Gomes et al. (2015a) measured the total drag of three sizes of kayak with three paddler weights (65, 75, and 85 kg) at 200, 500, and 1000 m race paces while towing the kayak across the water. Their results show small but important differences in

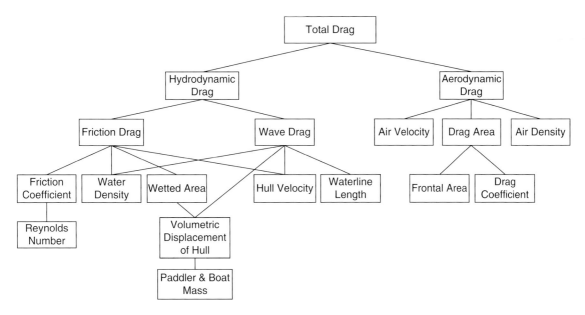

Figure 2.10 Factors that determine total drag. *Source*: Adapted from Jackson (1995). Reproduced with permission of Taylor & Francis.

Table 2.2 Values for the components of drag (N) and their relative contribution (%) to total drag for men's and women's kayak.

Men						
	K1		K2		K4	
Crew mass (kg)	81		162		324	
Boat mass (kg)	12		18		30	
Average velocity (m·s⁻¹)	4.83		5.41		5.49	
Drag	**(N)**	**(%)**	**(N)**	**(%)**	**(N)**	**(%)**
Friction drag	57.9	72	107.7	71	187.2	82
Wave drag	17.1	21	33.0	22	28.1	12
Air drag	5.6	7	410.5	7	14.5	6
Total drag	**80.6**		**151.2**		**229.8**	
Women						
	K1		K2		K4	
Crew mass (kg)	65		130		260	
Boat mass (kg)	12		18		30	
Average velocity (m·s⁻¹)	4.24		4.81		5.08	
Drag	**(N)**	**(%)**	**(N)**	**(%)**	**(N)**	**(%)**
Friction drag	41.4	73	78.5	73	146.7	83
Wave drag	10.9	19	20.9	19	17.2	10
Air drag	4.3	8	8.3	8	12.4	7
Total drag	**56.5**		**107.7**		**176.3**	

K1, Single kayak; K2, double kayak; K4, four-person kayak.
Source: Values are based upon those of Jackson (1995).

drag for the three kayak sizes and paddler masses, which have implications for the selection of the correct kayak size depending on paddler mass and boat velocity. Their directly measured values are generally are in line with the values determined by Jackson. It can be seen in Table 2.2 that friction drag has the largest contribution to total drag across all classes, followed by wave drag and then air drag. In reality, significant reductions in friction drag due to alterations in the friction coefficient may only be possible through significant changes in boat design. Given the constraints in the design and the development that have already taken place by manufacturers, this might not be possible, unless it is the scenario of a novice paddler moving from a more stable to less stable boat. Reductions in body mass would have an effect on both friction drag and wave drag, and Jackson (1995) states that a reduction in body mass of 3% would increase boat speed by 0.8%. Efforts targeting this as an intervention should be considered very carefully, however, due to the potentially negative effects on power production and general health.

A constant velocity is reached when the total drag forces equal the propulsive forces generated during the stroke. At this point, boat speed will only increase when the propulsive force increases, and again the boat speed will stabilize as the drag forces increase in response to the increased speed. The aim of any competitive paddler is to try to increase the average velocity over their chosen race distance. The options available to the paddler are to increase their physiological abilities to increase their rate of energy expenditure and power output, reduce their drag, or improve their paddling efficiency (something that will be covered further in this chapter).

As has been shown, drag is determined primarily by the shape of the boat and the mass of the boat and athlete. This drag is referred to as *passive drag*, which is due to the boat traveling in one fixed orientation without any deviation. However, there is also an additional *active drag* component caused during paddling as a result of the pitching, yawing, and rolling. It is not clear exactly how much active drag occurs at racing speeds, but Pendergast et al. (2005) measured the active drag component during kayaking at 3.0 m·s⁻¹ (a relatively slow pace) and

found that active drag was responsible for 14% of the total drag. Given the increased boat movements at race speeds, it is likely that the active drag component would be much larger.

In an earlier study, Pendergast et al. (1989) compared the drag of three different groups of athletes while paddling a slalom kayak and compared the total drag created by each group with the total drag created by the kayak moving at the same speed but without the paddler actually paddling (Figure 2.11). The lower skill level group created more active drag than the other two groups that consisted of experienced paddlers. The women's group produced less drag than the men due to their mass being on average 13 kg lighter. In support of this observation, Pendergast et al. (2005) followed a group of novice

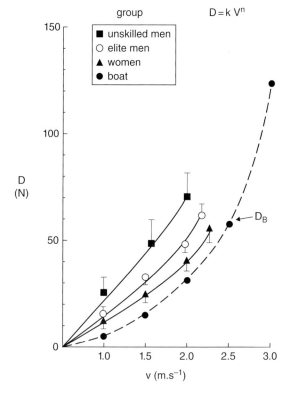

Figure 2.11 Drag (D) is plotted as a function of kayaking velocity (v). The dashed curve represents the drag of the boat carrying a kayaker who is not paddling (D_B). Solid lines represent the drag while paddling for each group. The difference between D_B and D for the different groups is the active drag. *Source*: Pendergast et al. (1989). Reproduced with permission of Springer.

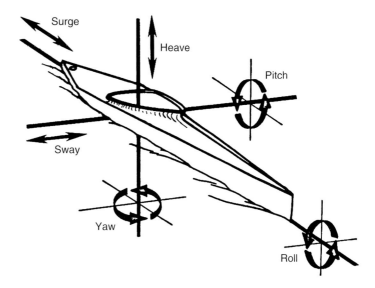

Figure 2.12 The movements of a boat. These are the same for a canoe. *Source*: Toro (1986).

sprint kayakers over a period of four years and found that their active drag while paddling at $3.0\,\mathrm{m\cdot s^{-1}}$ decreased by between 18 and 50% over this period as they accumulated more time in a kayak. It is clear that improved control of the boats' orientation during paddling will result in reduced total drag and an increased velocity for a given input.

As well as moving forward (surge), the effects of paddling cause the boat to yaw, pitch, roll, and heave (Figure 2.12). These resultant boat movements are created due to the movement of the body's center of mass during the stroke relative to the boat, and the lateral, vertical, and horizontal forces that are created by the paddle on the water during the paddle stroke. The paddle forces in each of these directions are highly changeable in magnitude and position relative to the boat during the stroke, and as such have differing effects upon the boat's movement (Table 2.3). The result of these movements is an increase in the friction drag and wave drag components, the magnitude of which is something that can be quite variable between different athletes of the same standard.

Mechanisms of propulsion

Propulsion when paddling is due to the creation of drag forces (using flat-bladed paddles) and lift forces as well as drag forces (using wing-style-bladed paddles) in kayaking. Figure 2.13 shows the

Table 2.3 Boat movements and their causes.

Pitching	Caused by forward and backward body movements during the stroke, and the direction of forces applied by the paddle, particularly at the end of the pull. Increases in pitch have a large effect on drag.
Rolling	Caused by the lateral movement of the center of mass in relation to the base of support (i.e. the seat and paddle, while the paddle is in the water).
Yawing	Caused by the off-center application of paddle forces. This can increase as the blade is moved away from the boat in kayaking. In canoeing, the yawing is kept to a minimum when the blade is kept close to the boat.
Heaving	Caused by the vertical movement of the center of mass during the stroke. More significant in canoeing during the transition from one stroke to the next.
Sway	The lateral movement of the boat during paddling. Most common in the K4.
Surge	This is desired movement as a direct result of paddle forces, and it can be modified by the forward and backward movement of the body during paddling.

K4, Four-person kayak.

relative differences in blade movement, with flat blades (applicable to flat kayaking blades and canoe blades) moving in a longitudinal direction close to the boat, and wing blades moving laterally as well as backward relative to the boat.

As the blade enters the water and forces are applied, a mass of water that is relative to the surface area of the blade is accelerated backward. The resulting drag force propels the boat forward via

(a) (b)

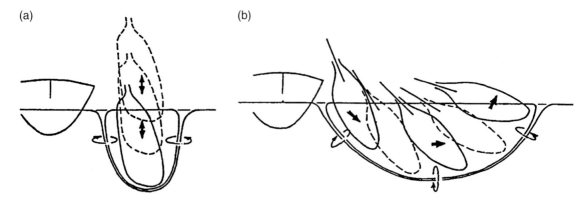

Figure 2.13 The path of the "flat" paddle (a) and "wing" paddle (b) in the water as viewed from the front. The difference in lateral movement is clearly seen. *Source*: Jackson (1995). Reproduced with permission of Taylor & Francis.

the hand, arm, torso, and connections with the hull via the seat and footrest. While this propulsive force drives the boat forward, there is a resulting blade slip, where the blade moves backward in the water as the drag forces are generated (Figure 2.14).

The drag force generated is determined primarily by the blade area and the velocity of the blade, and is described by the following equation:

$$F_d = \tfrac{1}{2}\rho A v^2 C_d$$

where F_d is the drag force, ρ is the fluid density, A the projected area of the blade, v the relative velocity between the blade and water, and C_d the coefficient of drag determined by the shape of the blade. The faster the blade movement relative to the water and the larger the blade size, the greater the propulsive forces. The force can also be moderated by the shape of the blade, although in reality the variations in shape between flat-bladed paddles have little effect on the generation of

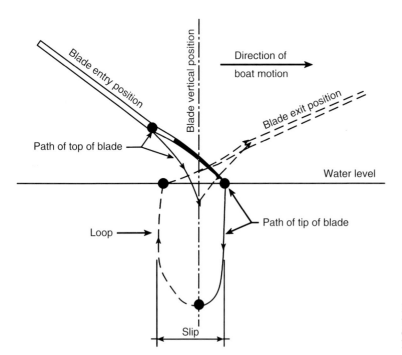

Figure 2.14 A sagittal plane view of the path of the paddle in the water during the stroke. *Source*: Fernandez-Nieves and de las Nieves (1998).

forces, and also by the water viscosity, which is mainly determined by water temperature. If everything else remains equal, forces will be higher in cold water compared to warm water. One of the unavoidable consequences of creating drag forces is that energy is given to the water in the form of velocity, which negatively affects paddling efficiency.

The wing-style blade generates a lateral movement due to its shape that results in a lift force being generated, and less blade slip for the same amount of propulsive force generated. The differences in lift and drag forces generated between blades were measured by Jackson et al. (1992), who determined that the wing blade had an efficiency of 89% compared to 75% of a flat blade. Large differences can be found in terms of both lateral movement and blade slip between individuals and even between left and right paddling sides in the same athlete. Figure 2.15 shows the difference in lateral movement and blade slip between two elite-level kayakers using wing-style paddles. In this example, kayaker A (solid line) has an initial forward movement of the blade relative to the water followed by a lateral movement. Crucially, less total blade slip occurs compared to kayaker B (dashed line), who demonstrated less lateral movement and greater blade slip.

The greater the blade slip, the larger the reduction in distance the boat would travel in that stroke if the blade did not slip in the water; therefore, the efficient paddler would minimize slip as much as possible to travel further with each stroke. Recent studies that have measured blade slip during race intensity efforts, during competitions, and of Olympic medal-winning athletes have ranged from 1 cm to as high as 33 cm per stroke. It has also been shown to vary in the stroke, with slip occurring at the beginning and end of the pull phase, but a forward movement of the paddle relative to the water (negative slip) occurring during the middle part of the pull phase when the blade is in a more vertical orientation. The relationship between blade slip and performance is not as clear as one might imagine, with high-level athletes often demonstrating significant amounts of blade slip. A complicating factor is that athletes can self-regulate the load on the blade, by reducing the amount of lateral blade movement or changing the orientation of the blade to reduce the propulsion-forming surface area. Both of these alterations will affect the magnitude of the blade slip, and may be constantly altered during a race to optimize velocity as fatigue occurs and the muscles' ability to generate force changes (Figure 2.16).

The orientation of the paddle relative to the water through the stroke is an important factor due to the resulting vertical and horizontal components of the force generated by the paddler. As can be seen in Figure 2.17, the horizontal component of force (F_H) is the propulsive force that moves the kayak forward, whereas the vertical component (F_V) will cause the bow of the kayak to lift at the catch, and the stern of the kayak to be pulled down at the exit. This vertical component and the resulting boat movement (pitching) will cause additional drag by altering the hull shape presented to the water, increasing form drag and therefore total drag.

In flat-bladed paddles such as those used in sprint canoes and in canoe slalom racing, propulsion is generated from drag forces alone, as lift forces are not created due to the shape of the blade. In these disciplines, the paddle is kept close to the side of the boat, and slip is minimized by careful selection of blade size and optimization of the stroke rate, although in comparison to

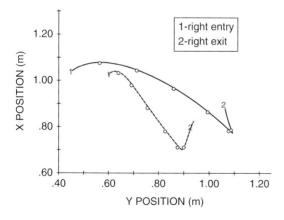

Figure 2.15 Plane view of the right blade tip path during the "pull phase" of the stroke in two elite kayakers. The right side of the kayak would be on the left side of the chart. *Source*: Kendal and Sanders (1992).

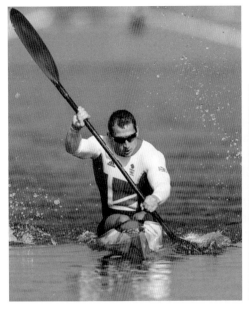
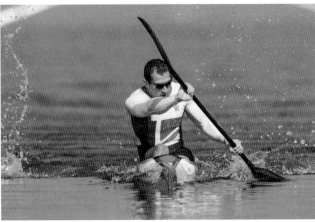

Figure 2.16 Images of Olympic champion Ed McKeever racing in the 200m final at the London Olympics. The lateral movement of the paddle during the pull phase can be clearly seen. *Source*: Balint Vekassy, © ICF.

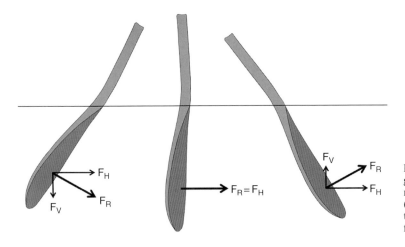

Figure 2.17 Components of generated force showing the resultant force (F_R), horizontal force (F_H), and vertical force (F_V). When the blade is vertical, the horizontal force is equal to the resultant force.

paddling with wing blades, slip is generally larger in comparative circumstances.

Propelling efficiency

The propelling efficiency (e_p) in paddling can be defined by the ratio of the power required to overcome drag (P_d) to the total power output produced (P_o), and can be explained by the following equation:

$$e_p = P_d/P_o$$

where the total power output is the sum of the power to overcome the drag forces present at that time and the power wasted in giving a kinetic energy change to the water. The kinetic energy

(KE) lost is determined by Newton's second law by the equation:

$$KE = \tfrac{1}{2}mv^2$$

where the velocity (v) is that given to the mass of the water (m) that is disturbed by the stroke. The larger the mass of water and the higher the velocity given to it, the greater the kinetic energy lost. Another method of increasing propelling efficiency is by reducing the forces required to overcome the boat's drag. This can be achieved by decreasing mass, or by reducing boat movements, in particular pitch, yaw, and heave. If the force generated by the contracting muscles is higher than the resistance of the blade and less than the resistance of the hull, the paddle will slip through the water, provide less propulsive force, and produce greater wasted kinetic energy.

Therefore, moving the wing blade a greater distance laterally and applying the same force to the paddle would result in the same propulsive force, less kinetic energy wasted, and a longer distance per stroke, as a result of less net slip, which also results in an increased propelling efficiency. The result would be paddling at the same speed but for a lower energy expenditure, which would have implications for either increasing maximal speed or sustaining a speed for a longer time period.

Paddling forces

A number of studies have reported the forces created by different groups of athletes paddling in various circumstances, but in general limited data exist. This is mainly due to the difficulty of measuring forces in the paddling environment without restricting the paddling movement. In an overview of applied sports biomechanics support in kayaking, Sperlich and Baker (2002) reported established norms for Australian national-level kayakers for two force-related variables. Peak force was 375 N for men and 290 N for women, and impulse 109 and 80 N·s for men and women, respectively. More recently, Gomes et al. (2015b), reported paddle forces in a group of national- and international-level male and female kayakers paddling at stroke rates from 60 to 124 (race pace) strokes per minute over 200 m. They reported peak forces ranging from 225 and 126 N at 60 strokes per minute to 274 and 153 N at 200 m race pace in males and females, respectively. These reported forces align well with the reported drag forces that occur while paddling, if allowing for a propelling efficiency that is less than 100%.

Figure 2.18 shows the paddle forces as well as the resulting boat movements from the left and right strokes while kayaking. This is fairly typical data from a high-level paddler that demonstrates large sustained high forces, clear phases of boat acceleration and deceleration, and some degree of asymmetry in force and acceleration. The paddle forces have been resolved into the vertical and horizontal components. Note that the paddle reaches the vertical position relatively early in the stroke, something that is not unusual, but has large implications for the magnitude of the vertical force component.

Note that there is some asymmetry between left and right strokes. The peak force is large on the right side, although the peak acceleration reached is larger on the left stroke. In fact, the horizontal impulse of the left stroke between A and C is 40.6 N·s versus 37.2 N·s on the right side. Blade slip is negligible on both strokes during this time. Therefore, the larger acceleration impulse and increased velocity on the left stroke are primarily due to the larger propulsive impulse. Note that the left stroke results in a net increase in velocity in comparison to the right, where the left stroke finishes at a greater velocity than it starts. The opposite happens in the right stroke, where the stroke finishes with a lower velocity than it starts.

Another feature seen in Figure 2.18 is that the paddle blade is vertical after approximately one-third of the total pull time, and a far larger proportion of the stroke time is spent with a paddle in an orientation that produces large vertical forces, causing the boat to pitch. The effects of paddle orientation on the vertical and horizontal forces can be seen in Figure 2.19, which is determined from the same data. These charts more clearly demonstrate the relationship between paddle orientation and force produced, and the magnitude of vertical force created (Figure 2.20).

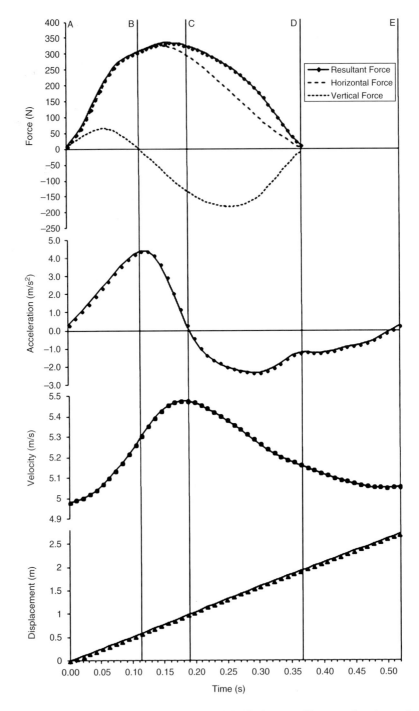

Figure 2.18 Typical average resultant, horizontal, and vertical paddle force, and boat acceleration, velocity, and displacement profiles, of 47 left-side strokes (left chart, page 26) and right-side strokes (right chart, page 27) from an international-level kayaker at 500 m race pace. The data shown are from the start of the stroke to the beginning of the next (opposite side) stroke. A, contact; B, paddle vertical; C, point of maximal kayak velocity; D, release; E, contact. Refer to Table 2.4 for an explanation of the key events.

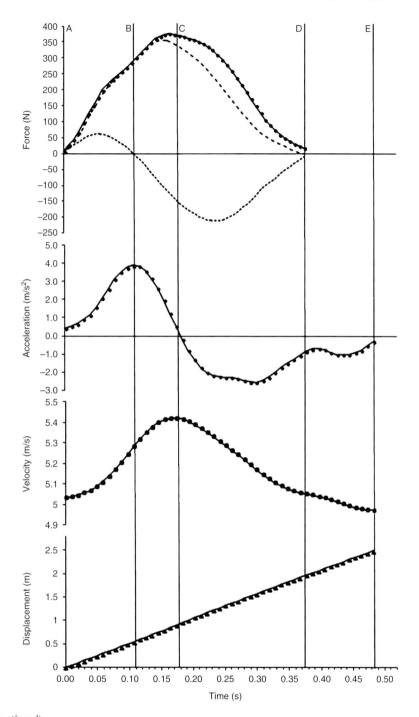

Figure 2.18 *(Continued)*

Table 2.4 Key events in the paddle stroke.

A	Point of first contact with the water	Paddle is usually at 40–50° to the water. A rapid increase in force production follows, which should result in a clear rapid increase in boat velocity. Due to the angle of the paddle, the horizontal force closely tracks the resultant force, and a small vertical force is present that causes the bow to lift (pitch).
B	The paddle is perpendicular to the water	In this position, all of the generated force is acting horizontally and is highly effective. Following this point, all forces continue to increase. Although the acceleration generally decreases, the velocity continues to rise.
C	Point when maximal velocity occurs	The point where the acceleration phase has ended and boat deceleration begins. Forces are still high, although normally peak force has occurred prior to this point, but not always. Vertical forces are high and increasing, which causes another period of boat pitching due to the blade pulling the boat downward. Note that in this next period, the negative acceleration is the largest despite the large paddle forces. The rate of deceleration decreases in line with the decrease in vertical force.
D	The paddle is released from the water and is transitioning from one stroke to the next in the aerial phase	Any changes to the negative acceleration from here are due to the movement of the body mass and in the hull profile caused by the necessary movement in preparation for the next stroke. Velocity decreases to a minimum just prior to the start of the next stroke.

Foot forces

The limited research on foot bar forces in kayaking has shown that the pushing forces on the footrest are generally higher than or equal to the forces found at the paddle, and are initiated immediately before the start of the paddle stroke. The paddling side foot pushes on the foot bar to move the same side pelvis backward by extending the leg. At the same time, the opposite side foot pulls against the foot strap or pull-bar (if used) to assist in the pelvis rotation on the seat. This synchronized movement of the pushing and pulling foot during the pull phase of the stroke helps increase the trunk rotation and the paddle force.

Research carried out by Begon et al. (2009) on a fully instrumented ergometer found that pelvis rotation, facilitated by the pushing actions of the lower limbs, contributes approximately 6% of the paddle propulsion forces. Recent research by Nilsson and Rosdahl (2016) has shown that when the legs are restricted in their extension and flexion, foot bar force and paddle force are reduced. They found decreases in paddle force of 21% and decreases in kayak speed of 16% in a group of five elite male kayakers when paddling at maximal effort when legs were restricted. This also supports other ergometer-based studies that show increases in paddle forces and ranges of movement due to the use of swivel seats. Caution must be used when evaluating studies on swivel seats, as the investigations to date were based on ergometers, and the outcomes have not been validated on water.

Performance-related factors

Temporal and phase analysis have been the most common methods used to analyze kayaking performance, as analysis of clearly identifiable elements of the stroke is relatively simple to achieve. Many investigators have examined the relationship between velocity and various phases of the stroke (Figure 2.21), and this has been summarized by McDonnell et al. (2013).

In applied practice, monitoring the relationships between stroke time, stroke distance, and velocity on an individual relationship has become popular and has led to an increasing use of GPS-type devices to measure velocity and stroke rate in training and racing. However, the roles of the subfactors that determine stroke time and stroke distance are not easily measured or understood, and as a result the identification of aspects of the stroke that should be altered to improve performance on an individual basis is not straightforward. To help in this process, a kayaking "deterministic" model has been developed by Wainwright et al. (2015) and can be used to help identify the various elements of a stroke cycle and understand how they interact to determine the average stroke velocity (Figure 2.22).

Stroke distance (distance traveled during the water and aerial phases) has not been shown to have a clear relationship with performance in the

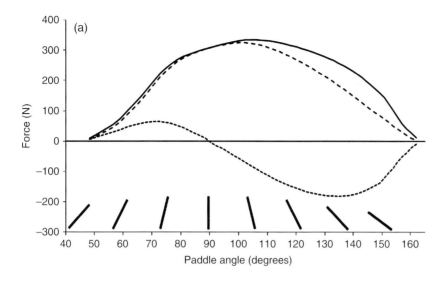

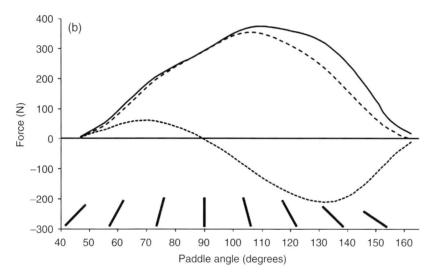

Figure 2.19 Left stroke (a) and right stroke (b) resultant (solid line), horizontal (dashed line), and vertical forces (dotted line) in relation to the sagittal plane paddle angles, which are illustrated on the chart.

studies that have examined it. For any given paddler, the general trend is that stroke distance decreases with increasing kayak velocity. High-level athletes tend to have a greater stroke distance for a given velocity and show a smaller rate of decrease in stroke distance as velocity increases. The relationship between velocity and stroke distance must be examined on an individual basis, as the relationship is often not straightforward. This can be seen in the deterministic model, where stroke distance

is determined by both the pull distance and the transition distance, with the pull distance determined by the stroke length (displacement of the paddle relative to the boat) and the blade slip. Therefore, it is not easy to try to make changes to stroke distance without knowing which of the sub-factors to modify.

Stroke time (duration of the water and aerial phases). This is more commonly converted to stroke rate (the number of single strokes in one minute), and

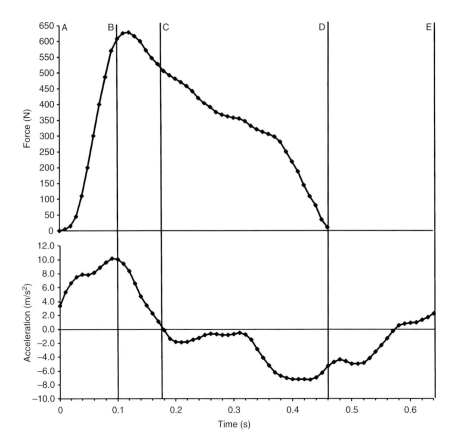

Figure 2.20 Typical average resultant paddle force and boat acceleration profiles of an international-level canoeist at 500 m race pace. The data shown are from the start of the stroke to the beginning of the next (opposite side) stroke. A, contact; B, paddle vertical; C, point of maximal canoe velocity; D, release; E, contact. Refer to Table 2.4 for an explanation of the key events.

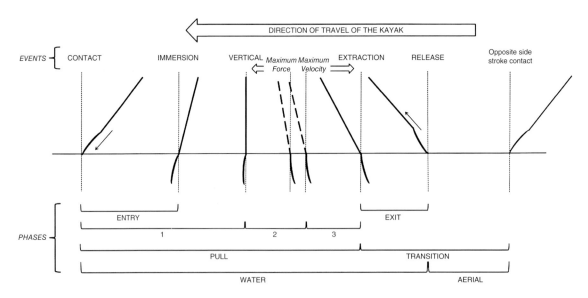

Figure 2.21 Events and phases of the kayak stroke. The exact position of the maximal force and maximal velocity varies with different styles and intensities of paddling, and can only be evaluated by monitoring the intrastroke velocity and paddle force profiles.

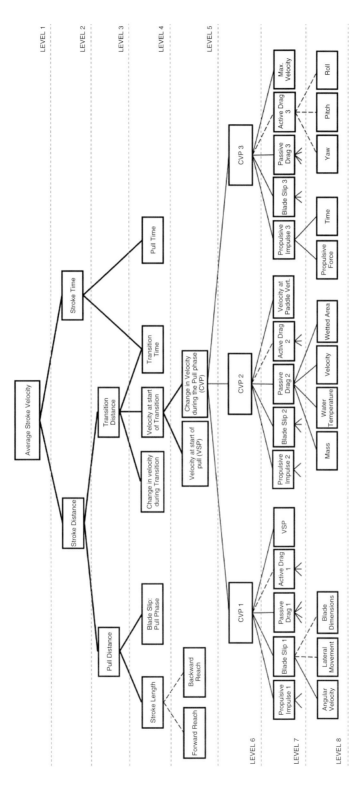

Figure 2.22 The kayaking deterministic model, from Wainwright et al. (2015). A deterministic model is a mechanical model where a factor on one level of the model is determined by the factors on the level immediately below it. By examining these relationships, an understanding of how each interact to alter factors within the model, and the cumulative effect on within-stroke velocity, can be gained.

generally has a strong relationship with velocity. Increases in stroke rate (i.e. a decrease in stroke time) normally create an increase in velocity, and the effect of increases in stroke rate is also moderated by the changes to stroke distance. The most common strategy that a kayaker uses to increase velocity is to increase stroke rate, but this is normally at the expense of some stroke distance. Stroke rates in the region of 130–150 strokes per minute are regularly recorded in 200 m racing.

As a result of a detailed analysis of on-water data using the deterministic model, a number of other key factors have been identified by Wainwright et al. (2015) that have a significant influence upon velocity.

Propulsive (horizontal) impulse. This is a key factor that creates an increase in the velocity during phases 1 and 2 (Figure 2.21) of the pull phase. It is created by the generation of large forces that act horizontally rather than the vertical forces that are directed downward and then upward (refer to Figures 2.17 and 2.18). The propulsive impulse plays a key role in accelerating the boat and increasing the velocity, and in general the majority of physical training that takes place is orientated toward increasing the capacity to create larger, sustainable impulses. However, it has been shown across a group of high-level kayakers that increases in propulsive impulses often only have a small effect on increasing the velocity within the pull phase of the stroke. As can be seen in the deterministic model, the propulsive impulse can be moderated by the blade slip. If the blade moves a long way backward in the water during the creation of the propulsive impulse, it generates a smaller increase in velocity than if there was little or no blade slip, for example. The paddler should aim to increase their ability to produce large propulsive impulses, but equal attention should be paid to aspects of technique that impact the effectiveness of the propulsive impulse generated (i.e. minimizing blade slip).

Paddle angle (sagittal plane/side view). The orientation of the paddle plays a critical role in the effectiveness of the paddle force and the impulse. In the early part of the stroke (Figure 2.17), the majority of the force applied is horizontal force, with a small proportion going to the creation of a vertical force. However, once the paddle is past the vertical position, which in many athletes occurs relatively early

in the stroke, the vertical force starts to increase rapidly. Although the horizontal forces remain high, the effect of the increasing vertical forces is to create a pitching movement of the boat, which acts to slow the boat. The impact of the vertical forces on boat acceleration and velocity can be seen in Figure 2.18, where the boat starts to decelerate approximately halfway through the pull phase. This is a very common chain of events, and the longer the paddle can create forces prior to the vertical position, the more effective any generated force is. The magnitude of the vertical and horizontal forces created relative to the resultant force can be moderated by changing the paddle angle during the pull phase.

Blade slip. Both the pull distance and the effectiveness of the propulsive impulse are moderated by the blade slip, which should be minimized where possible and appropriate. Blade slip appears to be more likely to occur when the paddle is at smaller and larger angles such as those found at the beginning (phase 1) and end (phase 3) of the pull phase. Negative blade slip, where the paddle moves forward in the water as it moves laterally (as a result of large lift forces), has been found to occur during the middle (phase 2) of the pull phase where the blade is in a more vertical orientation. It is likely that the lateral blade movement, which would be greatest during phase 2, is related to the forward displacement of the blade during this period.

Change in velocity during the transition. Examination of the deterministic model shows that the transition distance is determined by the duration of this phase, the velocity at the start of the phase, and the change in velocity during the phase. The first two factors are relatively obvious and controlled by other aspects of the stroke, but the change in velocity has been shown to be variable within paddlers and can also have a strong influence upon the transition distance. Although little formal research has been carried out to identify what aspects of the kayaking movement lead to larger or smaller decreases in velocity and therefore distance, it is clear that boat movements that cause changes in the drag are primarily responsible. Efforts should be made to keep the boat movements, which are likely to have been caused during the pull phase, to a minimum during the transition to optimize the distance traveled during the transition time.

Stroke length. The position that the blade enters the water and the position relative to the position of entry that the blade leaves the water determine the stroke length. It is something that is relatively easily controlled by the athlete while paddling, and changes in the stroke length determine the pull distance along with the blade slip. The longer the stroke length, the further the boat will travel during the pull phase, as long as the blade slip is kept constant. However, due to the negative effects of producing forces toward the end of the stroke, attention should be made to enter the paddle further forward rather than further backward. Although this may lead to an increase in vertical forces, as can been seen in Figure 2.18, the potential for these to become large enough to cause significant negative effects is relatively small. Attention should be paid to seat height, paddle length, and trunk rotation as these factors can all influence the position of blade entry (contact) with the water.

When traveling in a straight line in kayaking and canoeing (and slalom in this example), there are three fundamental events that take place, which the kayaker must try to optimize for the task:

1 To enable the boat to travel as far as possible while the paddle is in the water (i.e. a large pull distance)
2 To increase the velocity of the boat during the pull phase in order that the velocity is as high as possible at the end of the pull phase (i.e. a large change in velocity during the pull)
3 To minimize the decrease in velocity during the transition phase (i.e. minimize the change in velocity during the transition).

The paddler achieves these without really being aware of it, but in most cases these events are not optimized. This is not surprising given the number of factors involved and the complexity of their interaction (as shown in the deterministic model). The paddler also alters the time duration of each of the phases so that more or less time can be given to each depending upon the goal of the task. For example, the transition time may be reduced to prevent an excessive decrease in velocity, with relatively more time given to increase the stroke length, which increases the stroke distance, creates a larger propulsive impulse in the early phases of the stroke, and increases the velocity within the pull phase. There is a complex chain of events that takes place that eventually has an impact upon the boat's velocity, and it is the nature of this complexity that means that it is not always that easy to detect the impact of small technique interventions.

Equipment setup

Our knowledge of optimal equipment setup based upon an individual's physical characteristics is limited. Some research has taken place that helps reaffirm a general understanding that limb lengths and athlete height play a role in the choice of paddle length. However, identification of the key factors involved and their interrelationships in the optimization of the setup of equipment is not complete. Measures of a number of competitors (11 females and 31 males) at the Sydney Olympic Games (Ong et al. 2005) have gone some way to establish some norms for this athlete group. The average values for the key measurements can be found in Table 2.5.

Paddle grip width (PGW) as a percentage of total paddle length was found to be 33.0 and 31.5% for males and females, respectively, on average. The study also found the foot bar–to-seat distance (FBD) and PGW (distance between index fingers) to be related to body height. The authors proposed the following setup based upon their findings:

$$FBD(cm) = 15.975 + (0.603 \times Height)$$

$$PGW(cm) = 3.557 + (0.376 \times Height)$$

Table 2.5 Average values for equipment measures in sprint kayakers (in centimeters).

	Men	Women
Athlete height	184.5	168.6
Seat height (floor to lowest point on the seat)	20.8	20.5
Foot bar distance (horizontal distance from lowest point of seat to middle of foot bar)	94.9	87.2
Paddle length (horizontal distance between blade tips)	220.2	215.3
Paddle grip width (distance between the index fingers when paddles are held normally)	72.8	67.9

Source: From Ong et al. (2005).

Caution must be used when applying these suggested formulae, as the authors of this study found that when these were applied to paddlers, it did not always result in an improvement in performance. It is likely that there are additional factors that were not measured that determine an optimum PGW and footrest setup for each paddler. However, the equations may be a starting point from which to base further individualized adjustments.

CANOE SLALOM

Equipment

Equipment changes in canoe slalom (see Table 2.6) were often driven by rule changes and course changes. The course length changed from one that took approximately 265 seconds in the 1960s to 205 seconds in the 1970s and 1980s. By 2015, rac-

Table 2.6 Major events in the development of equipment in canoe slalom.

1949	First World Championships held in Geneva. Folding-style boats were the boat of choice.
1950s	Bicycle-style helmets used for paddling helmets. Initial buoyancy aids were made using car-tire inner tubes.
1960s	Fiberglass boats first started to be used in competitions, starting with the C2 class. Folding-style boats became phased out. "Wilde" fiberglass helmets from Czechoslovakia were predominantly used rather than the leather bicycle-style designs. Harishok developed the first air-filled sport-specific buoyancy aid, which was later improved with the use of closed-cell foam.
1970s	Fiberglass paddles started to be introduced. Until this point, they were wooden with aluminum tips. Lower volume boats were first used at the Munich Olympics for racing on the Augsburg Eiskanal, a design trend that was started by the DDR team. Rule changes enable the bows and sterns of boats to be lower than the decks. This influenced techniques that were used to negotiate gates. The larger scale of manufacturing of slalom boats improved accessibility to higher quality boats; prior to this, boats were essentially homemade using shared molds. Kevlar boats were used by the USA team at the World Championships in Switzerland in 1973. A new "close-cockpit" C2 is raced by Johnny Evans (representing the USA) at the World Championships in Yugoslavia in 1975. Lettmann introduced the "Perfekt" kayak, a revolution in design until it was later banned due to the ends being dangerously narrow (Figure 2.24). Plastic helmets were developed and started to replace fiberglass due to being more robust.
1980s	Crankshaft paddles were introduced in the early 1980s, and were used by Richard Fox in particular. There became a split in boat design as boats started to become more specialized for slalom or downriver racing. Pole heights increased to 15 cm above the water, which led to an increased volume and depth in the bows of boats. Minimum weight rules were introduced to ensure boats were of robust construction. Minimum bow and stern radius (of 2 cm horizontally and 1 cm vertically, respectively) rule was introduced for safety reasons. Adjustable footrests were introduced for kayaks.
1990s	Hull shape changed from having rounded sides to having more vertical sides. Kayak paddle "feather" angles decreased from the traditional 90° to improve wrist comfort. Kayak paddles in particular became more asymmetric and scooped to improve effectiveness. Boats and paddles were increasingly constructed using carbon–kevlar and carbon.
2000s	Boat lengths reduced to 3.5 m from 4.0 m after the Athens Olympics, facilitating faster turns that were important following the trend to shorter, more technical course designs. Pole heights increased further to 20 cm above the water, leading to tighter turns around upstream gates.
2010s	Boat fittings increasingly individualized using laser-cut high-density foam or carbon-molding processes. Kayak "hull-fins" introduced and used by an increasing number of athletes. Minimum weights for boats increased to 9 kg for K1/C1 and 15 kg for C2.

C1, Single canoe; C2, double canoe; DDR, East Germany; K1, single kayak; K2, double kayak; K4, four-person kayak.

ing times for the men's kayak class often dropped to below 90 seconds. Gate penalties were initially reduced from 20 to 10 seconds in 1979, to five seconds in 1981, and then to two seconds in 1997. The use of natural rivers has made way to an increased use of artificial courses for major competitions, with the last major canoe slalom championship race on a natural river being held on the Isère River at Bourg-Saint-Maurice, France, in 2002. The decreased gate penalties and the shorter courses with more consistent water have led to the importance of tighter and faster turns being a key driver for boat design across the classes. The choice of boat an athlete makes and the relative position of the seat are still very much determined through a process of subjective feedback from the athlete, combined with comparisons of split times taken over repeated sections of a course to indicate differences in performance. Although the majority of boats used are production boats from the major canoe slalom manufacturers, athletes at the top end of the discipline often work with the manufacturers to make small customizations to the shape to suit their own paddling style (Figures 2.23–2.25).

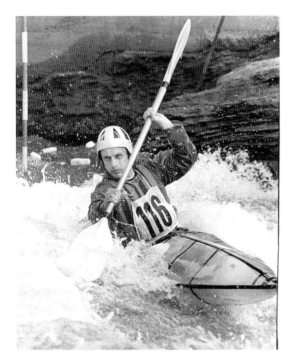

Figure 2.23 John MacLeod (representing Great Britain) paddling at Zwickau, Germany, circa 1971. As was typical of the era, equipment was self-developed and manufactured. In this case, the kayak was homemade with a fiberglass resin and carbon construction, and paddles were homemade consisting of fiberglass and resin blades and titanium shafts. *Source*: Courtesy of John MacLeod.

Biomechanics

Fluid mechanics

The interaction between the boat and water is very different in canoe slalom. At times, the athlete is working against the direction of the flow of the water to reach a particular gate or get through a water feature, whereas at other times the flow and direction of water are being used to propel the boat on the course. Therefore, minimizing the drag forces is very important on some sections of the course, whereas at other times the drag forces are less important. At higher competitive levels of the sport, there is an increasing proportion of a race where the athlete must move their boat faster than the speed of the water if they are to be successful, and in these circumstances a greater emphasis is

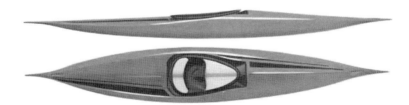

Figure 2.24 Lettmann Perfekt. Gaybo Ltd. catalog, 1976. The boat has a full fiberglass construction and material taken out of the ends to aid faster turns. The bow and stern are very narrow, which led to this design being banned later on safety grounds. *Source*: Courtesy of Lettmann GmbH.

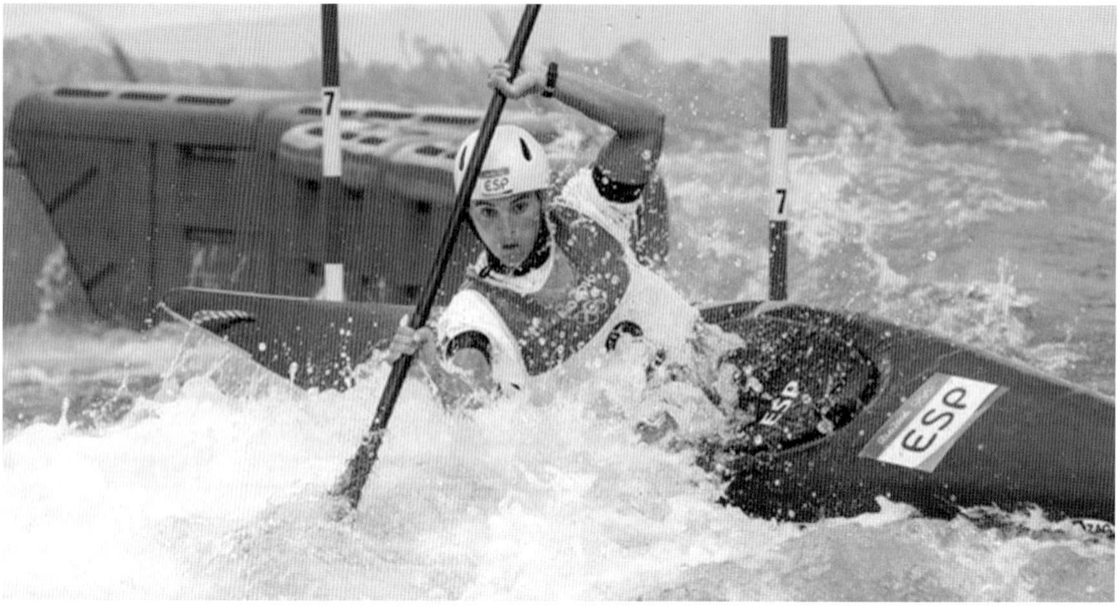

Figure 2.25 Maialen Chourraut (representing Spain) on her gold medal–winning run at the Rio 2016 Olympics. Note the high-volume front deck area and the low-volume rear deck. The helmet is a lightweight plastic model, and there is a sport-specific low-volume buoyancy aid. The tight-fitting neoprene spraydeck ensures virtually no water enters the boat. The paddle as well as canoe are constructed of carbon fiber. *Source*: Balint Vekassy, © ICF.

placed upon achieving a smaller drag either through boat design or the weight of the paddler and his equipment. The results of the study by Pendergast et al. (1989) (Figure 2.11) demonstrate the importance of paddling skill as a means of reducing drag in canoe slalom. When paddling on whitewater, the athlete can also change the boat's shape with respect to the direction of the water flow by altering the boat's orientation. This can be achieved primarily by moving the body's center of mass relative to the boat, and the change in orientation of the boat can significantly alter the boat's characteristics, making it easier to turn, grip the water, or even pop out of the water using the inherent buoyancy of the boat's volume. It is the skill of the athlete to use the three-dimensional shape of the boat to suit the immediate needs on the whitewater at any time.

Paddle forces

Very little information has been published on the paddle forces created during canoe slalom on white-

water. Some early work, primarily carried out by Juergen Sperlich (for example, Sperlich and Klauk 1992), showed peak forces in the region of 500 N for a kayak repeating a four-gate sequence. Further measurements of paddling on whitewater carried out by the author have shown that applied forces are highly variable and intermittent in nature, with peak forces of up to 600 N depending upon the athlete in question, the force of the water, the orientation of the gate, and the technique selected. An example of the forces is shown in Figure 2.26. Average peak forces for a full slalom run would normally be in the region of 300–350 N for men's kayaks, 250–300 N for women's kayaks, and 350–400 N for men's canoes.

While the ability to generate large rapid forces in canoe slalom is important, so is the ability to use them effectively. Forces are used not only for propelling the boat forward, but also for turning and steering. Highly skilled slalom paddlers are able to minimize the use of their strokes at maximum force by using the water effectively and only using their maximal force at key times on the run, such as when rectifying mistakes or maintaining

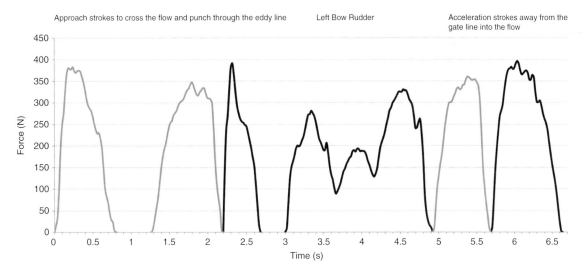

Figure 2.26 Paddle forces generated to complete a left-hand upstream gate on whitewater (black lines: left-hand forces; gray lines: right-hand forces). Note that the approach strokes are variable in force and timing due to the athlete making final adjustments to the approach speed and angle. The strokes after exiting the gate are normally large and rapid to accelerate the kayak. Note the duration and variation in the bow-rudder stroke as the athlete makes adjustments to maintain the speed and position of the kayak as it turns around the gate pole.

velocities through particularly draggy parts of the course. By using maximal capacities sparingly, and reducing resistance where possible, fatigue is offset, and higher levels of coordination and skill can be executed over the whole run.

Although there is a large variation in the types of strokes used during a single run on a whitewater course, the same principles described for effective paddle strokes in sprint racing apply in canoe slalom. Due to the relatively flat shape of the blades used, no lift forces are generated, so the basic forward stroke should be kept close to the side of the boat to minimize the yawl effect. An excellent online "Technique Library" that provides video examples of a large number of the key techniques used on whitewater can be found at www.slalomtechnique.co.uk.

Racing strategies

The tactics and strategies used in canoe slalom competitions to negotiate the course as fast as possible are very much in the coaching domain and are determined by the athlete and coach in the hours before each run takes place once the gate configuration has been finalized. Recently, a study by Hunter (2009) investigated how the path taken by national team kayaks and canoes to negotiate an upstream gate influenced the time taken. The study showed that there was a strong correlation between the time taken and the distance to the inside pole during the exit from the gate, and suggested that paddlers should focus upon minimizing the distance between their head and the inside pole to improve performance. When analyzing the path taken by the fastest and slowest boats, it was found that the two slowest boats in each category took a tighter line leading into the gate, but their position then became wider and further past the gate line than the position of the fastest boats (Figure 2.27). This suggests that the approach toward the gate as well as the execution around the gate are important for faster times.

Equipment setup

There has been little investigation of the equipment and its setup for slalom paddlers, but a study by Ong et al. (2005) did go some way to describe

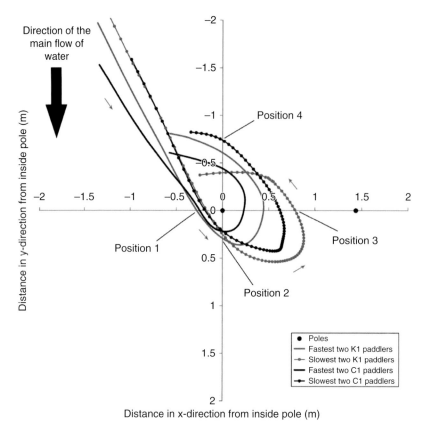

Figure 2.27 Boat trajectories of slalom C1s and K1s while negotiating an upstream gate. The fastest C1s and K1s exhibited a wider approach and kept closer to the inside pole. *Source*: Hunter (2009). Reproduced with permission of Taylor & Francis.

Table 2.7 Average values for equipment measures in slalom kayakers (in centimeters).

	Men	**Women**
Athlete height	177.1	166.7
Seat height (floor to lowest point on the seat)	21.7	20.9
Foot bar distance (horizontal distance from lowest point of seat to middle of foot bar)	88.1	84.7
Paddle length (horizontal distance between blade tips)	203.0	199.5
Paddle grip width (distance between the index fingers when paddles are held normally)	70.3	66.3

Source: From Ong et al. (2005).

the setup of some of the equipment of 12 male and 12 female Olympic slalom kayak paddlers. They measured paddle setup as well as foot bar distance and seat height (Table 2.7).

These values only represent a small population of Olympic paddlers, and may not be representative of the whole sport. While these values may provide an indication for kayak paddlers, no data were reported for the C1 or double canoe (C2) classes. The average PGW as a percentage of total paddle length was 34.6 and 33.2% in males and females, respectively, which may also be used as a guide for setting up paddles irrespective of length.

Bibliography

Begon, M., Colloud, F., and Lacouture, P. (2009). Measurement of contact forces on a kayak ergometer with a sliding footrest-seat complex. *Sports Engin* 11: 67–73.

Fernandez-Nieves, A. and de las Nieves, F.J. (1998). About the propulsive system of a kayak and of Basiliscus Basiliscus. *Eur J Physics* 19: 425–429.

Gomes, B.B., Conceição, F.A.V., Pendergast, D.R., Sanders, R.H., Vaz, M.A.P., and Vilas-Boas, J.P. (2015a) Is passive drag dependent on the interaction of kayak design and paddler weight in flat-water kayaking? *Sports Biomech*, 14, 394–403. doi: https://doi.org/10.1080/14763141.2015.1090475

Gomes, B.B., Ramos, N.V. Conceição, F.A.V., Sanders, R.H., Vaz, M.A.P., and Vilas-Boas, J.P. (2015b) Paddling force profiles at different stroke rates in elite sprint kayaking. *J Appl Biomech*, 31, 258–263. doi: https://doi.org/10.1123/jab.2014-0114

Hunter, A. (2009) Canoe slalom boat trajectory while negotiating an upstream gate. *Sports Biomech*, 8(2), 105–113. doi: https://doi.org/10.1080/14763140902934837

Jackson, P.S. (1995). Performance prediction for Olympic kayaks. *J Sports Sci* 13: 239–245.

Jackson, P.S., Locke, N., and Brown, P. (1992) The hydrodynamics of paddle propulsion. Paper presented at the 11th Australasian Fluid Mechanics conference, Hobart, Australia.

Kendal, S.J. and Sanders, R.H. (1992). The technique of elite flatwater kayak paddlers using the wing paddle. *Intl J Sport Biomech* 8: 233–250.

McDonnell, L.K., Hume, P.A., and Nolte, V. (2013). A deterministic model based on evidence for the associations between kinematic variables and sprint kayak performance. *Sports Biomech* 12 (3): 205–220.

Nilsson, J.E., and Rosdahl, H.G. (2016) Contribution of leg muscle forces to paddle force and kayak speed during maximal effort flat-water paddling. *Intl J Sports Physiol Perform*, 11(1): 22–27. doi: https://doi.org/10.1123/ijspp.2014-0030

Ong, K.B., Ackland, T.R., Hume, P.A. et al. (2005). Equipment set-up among Olympic sprint and slalom kayak paddlers. *Sports Biomech* 4: 47–58.

Pendergast, D.R., Bushnell, D., Wilson, D.W., and Cerretelli, P. (1989). Energetics of kayaking. *Eur J Appl Physiol* 59: 342–350.

Pendergast, D., Mollendorf, J., Zamparo, P. et al. (2005). The influence of drag on human locomotion in water. *Undersea Hyperbaric Med* 32: 45–57.

Sperlich, J. and Baker, J. (2002). Biomechanical testing in elite canoeing. In: *Scientific proceedings of the 20th International Symposium on Biomechanics in Sports* (ed. J.E. Gianikellis), 44–47. Caceres, Spain: University of Extremadura.

Sperlich, J., and Klauk, J. (1992) Biomechanics of canoe slalom: measuring techniques and diagnostic possibilities. In: Rodano, R., Ferringo, G., and Santambrogio, G.C. (eds.), *Scientific proceedings of the 10th International Symposium of Biomechanics in Sports*, Milan, pp. 82–84.

Toro, A. (1986). *Canoeing: An Olympic sport*. San Francisco, CA: Olympian Graphics.

Wainwright, B.G., Cooke, C.B., and Low, C. (2015) Performance related technique factors in Olympic Sprint kayaking. In: *Scientific proceedings of the 33rd International Conference on Biomechanics in Sports*. Poitiers, France: University of Poitiers.

Chapter 3
The canoe/kayak athlete

Petra Lundström[1], Jorunn Sundgot Borgen[2], and Don McKenzie[3]

[1]Department of Molecular Medicine and Surgery, Karolinska Institute, Solna, Sweden

[2]Department of Sports Medicine, Norwegian School of Sports Sciences, Oslo, Norway

[3]Division of Sport and Exercise Medicine, The University of British Columbia, Vancouver, BC, Canada

Physical structure as well as technique, fitness, psychology, and race strategy are essential factors for winning a race. Paddling requires high values for maximal aerobic and anaerobic capacities in combination with a high upper-body and trunk musculature as well as strength. This is regardless of being female or male. Many functional differences between male and female athletes are the result of basic differences in body size and body composition. Because cellular mechanisms that control the physiological and biochemical responses to exercise are not identical for both genders, it is clear that slightly different quantitative responses can result in significant performance differences.

Data from anthropometric measurements in recent decades, on male and female elite canoe/kayak paddlers, report less body fat and increased upper-body and arm musculature that is related to performance and more successful paddling. However, the energy needs in terms of cholesterol (CHO), protein, fat, and a combination of macronutrients are basically the same, expressed as gram per kilogram of body weight. Therefore, it is of great importance for both coaches and athletes to understand the differences in physiological and nutritional requirements between genders.

More physiological and performance-related data have been reported for male competitive paddlers than for their female counterparts. However, there are gender differences, particularly due to menstruation, and training during pregnancy as well as after birth are issues specific to female athletes. This portion of the chapter will focus on female athlete–specific issues in paddlers.

Body composition: a performance variable

Body composition and anthropometry play an important role for athletic performance in paddling. In general, men and women have different body compositions, specifically more fat-free mass in males and more fat mass in women after puberty due to different hormonal status. However, in elite athletes, these variables may change related to sport-specific physiological demands, thus making women leaner with lower fat mass and more fat-free mass than the general female reference body composition. Sport-specific references in body composition exist in some sports, but they should be carefully interpreted and communicated, especially to the young female athlete. The reference models should not be used as a goal to achieve the perfect sport-specific body composition, due to the fact that fat mass and fat-free mass depend on not only the type of sport and its specific training and nutritional demands. Other factors such as age, genetics, and differences in race and ethnicity also are of major importance. However, there is little doubt that being leaner is an advantage in a number of sports, and this is also true in paddling sports. It is therefore a desire to optimize performance by improving the power-to-weight ratio also in female paddlers. International-level female paddlers have a body composition with a greater than average proportional thigh length, greater than average shoulder and chest breadths, and proportionally larger upper-body girths.

Kayak, canoe, and slalom racing is performed on water. While a larger individual may have a larger absolute peak oxygen consumption (VO_2), potentially, a too large body mass of the paddler may also negatively affect the relative peak VO_2 attainable for propelling the boat. The increased weight will cause the boat to sit deeper in the water, increasing wetted area, total frictional resistance, and wave drag, thereby increasing the resistance that must be overcome by the paddler to propel the boat forward.

Although suggestions for optimal body fat content for various sports may be found in some textbooks, none of these are evidence-based. Given the variability between individuals and the errors inherent in assessment of body fat content, it seems unlikely that a single critical value can ever be identified. Nonetheless, the values stated in the literature may serve as a useful guide. It is recommended that an athlete measures body composition during the in- and off-season on a regular basis, to track the individual changes and how they are related to health, adaptation to training, and performance. For those athletes who need guidance for optimizing energy and nutrient intake and/or for weight loss or change in body composition, the IOC Medical Commission has developed excellent guidelines.

Energy metabolism and measurements

Paddling, regardless of events, is a sport that involves mainly a high maximal aerobic power, but also the anaerobic energy system is included to attain a successful performance. The sport requires

high energy availability to achieve a high metabolic rate (e.g. a high capacity to produce adenosine triphosphate [ATP] to match the energy need of the working muscle). This is attainable when energy intake and energy expenditure equal over time, maintaining a balanced energy intake. The challenge for an athlete involved in such an energy-demanding sport as paddling is to match the energy costs with sufficient energy intake. Hormones involved in appetite regulation as well as the reward system in the brain could precede satiety without actually covering the energy costs. Over time, even a small deficit can negatively affect basal physiological functions, health, and performance.

To estimate an athlete's energy demand, it is necessary to have a knowledge of daily total energy expenditure (TEE) and the resting metabolic rate (RMR). TEE is the most variable factor, while RMR is the largest. RMR depends on the total metabolic activity of all organs in the body. The current standard equations, recommended by the American College of Sports Medicine (ACSM), have not, however, been validated in an athletic population.

Therefore, predictions of RMR as well as TEE must be used cautiously. Studies have shown that predicted equations overestimate RMR in female athletes. Therefore, advice to elite athletes always has to be based on observations in the individual athlete.

Body composition, carbohydrate intake, and rapid weight loss

In recent decades, it has become popular to lose weight by reducing the CHO intake. Therefore, in some athletes, it could be tempting to reduce body weight rapidly by reducing the CHO intake. It has to be stressed that all rapid weight loss always involves a loss of fat-free mass (including skeletal muscle) as well as body fat. Over the long term, if frequently repeated, this will negatively affect RMR, body composition, and ultimately health and performance.

The importance of CHO in sport nutrition stands in contrast to the fact that CHO is regarded as the main cause of the increasing obesity epidemic worldwide. It is well established that when the glycogen stores have reached their full capacity, the eventual excess sugar is converted and stored as fat. Overconsumption of CHO is as bad as underconsumption. It must be emphasized that the main source of CHO shall be regular foods, but during periods of hard training or competition, bars, gels, dried fruits, juices, and sport drinks are good sources for extra CHO.

Relative energy deficiency

While some female athletes find it easy to achieve an optimal body composition, many athletes do not and may get confused in trying to balance energy and nutritional needs. The balance between the goal to reach the optimal body composition and at the same time sustain high training loads, optimizing recovery and performance, is difficult. Especially, young female athletes endeavoring to achieve body composition goals might experience low energy deficiency. Recently, an expert group from the IOC called attention to a problem that is wider and more complex than that originally identified as the *Female Athlete Triad*. The expert group introduced a broader, more comprehensive term: *Relative Energy Deficiency in Sport* (RED-S). The cause of RED-S is the scenario termed *low energy availability* (LEA), where an individual's dietary energy intake is insufficient to support the energy expenditure required for health, function, and daily living, once the costs of exercise and sporting activities are taken into account. RED-S refers to impaired physiological functioning caused by relative energy deficiency, and it includes but is not limited to impairments of metabolic rate, menstrual function, bone health, immunity, protein synthesis, and cardiovascular health. Athletes, coaches, and healthcare staff should know that athletes who suffer from long-term RED-S may develop nutrient deficiencies (including anemia), chronic fatigue, and increased risk of infections and illnesses. Physiological and medical complications may involve many organ systems. Psychological stress and/or depression can also result in LEA and eating disorders.

The hormone estrogen is a main regulator of the female reproductive system and is also involved as a regulator in other organ systems, such as the growth and maturation of bone in young females and bone turnover in adult women.

LEA may induce suppression of the hypothalamic–pituitary–ovarian axis with a state of estrogen deficiency as well as alteration in thyroid hormone regulation. The positive exercise-induced response on bone mass and skeletal health may be jeopardized if amenorrhea is present, particularly in non-weight-bearing sports such as paddling. Estrogen deficiency may modify energy balance by decreasing RMR and spontaneous physical activity. Taken together, estrogen deficiency over time could have detrimental effects on health and ultimately performance.

Calcium and vitamin D

Calcium is an ion that has a crucial role in many physiological processes. More than 90% of calcium is found in bones, where it provides hard tissue with its strength. Extracellular levels are rigorously regulated, and bone tissue serves as a reservoir for calcium. The challenge is to maintain a constant level of calcium in serum and, at the same time, provide adequate amounts to keep up bone strength and other processes. Decreases in calcium homeostasis are done by activating bone resorption, reducing urinary calcium excretion, and increasing intestinal absorption of calcium. Little is known about the intake of calcium in female athletes. However, athletes who are trying to decrease their weight might have substandard intake, and circumscribed data suggest that amenorrheic athletes have an increased need of calcium ($500\,mg\cdot day^{-1}$) to maintain calcium balance due to estrogen deficiency. The most acknowledged source of calcium is dairy products. Other sources are green vegetables, fruits, legumes, eggs, and meat.

Vitamin D serves as a regulator of calcium exchange of the gut, bone, and the renal tubule, and it has an important function in strengthening bone and repairing microfractures that might occur during heavy workloads. Another important function is in relation to the immune system. The severity and frequency of upper respiratory tract infections in the winter months seem to be related to vitamin D. Concentrations $>75\,nmol\cdot l^{-1}$ appear to be beneficial. Vitamin D deficiency has been described in athletes and is a problem especially in female athletes with estrogen deficiency. The prevalence of deficiency varies by sport, geographic location, and skin color. Whether paddlers are exposed to sufficient sunlight is not known. Dietary assessments have found that athletes do not meet the dietary recommendations in many countries. Athletes who are at risk are those with low consumption of dairy products and a high intake of fiber-rich foods that might decrease the absorption in the gut.

Iron and performance in female paddlers

Iron deficiency, if associated with true anemia (and not just sports anemia, as discussed further in this section), may be associated with several performance-related symptoms such as fatigue and impaired aerobic endurance capacity. Iron is essential for basic biochemical activities such as energy metabolism, and true deficiency of iron with anemia significantly decreases oxygen transport capacity by decreasing total hemoglobin (Hb) volume.

Iron deficiency is common among female athletes, especially in endurance sports. A number of factors, including heavy or frequent menstrual bleeding, low energy intake, vegetarian choice of foodstuffs, gastrointestinal bleeding, exercise-dependent transient inflammatory response (interleukin-6 [IL6], a cytokine released from contracting muscle, increases the risk of iron depletion, particularly in glycogen-depleted situations), injuries, and medication (such as anti-inflammatory drugs), may affect iron status.

The mechanism behind so-called "sports anemia" is an increase in plasma volume due to post-exercise plasma volume expansion after periods of intense physical activity. When plasma volume increases relatively more than the red blood cell volume, there will be a relative decrease in hematocrit and Hb concentration (i.e. sports anemia) despite an increase in the total volume of red blood cells.

Iron deficiency should always be diagnosed by a physician. Iron supplements in combination with dietary intervention are recommended as treatment. It is also advisable to analyze iron stores before training or competing at high altitude, since a depleted iron store will negatively affect adaptation and performance and increase the risk of infections. It must, however, be emphasized that iron supplements will enhance performance in individuals who have true iron deficiency anemia, but not in athletes with normal iron stores (even though Hb concentration might be low due to sports anemia).

Menstrual dysfunction

The onset of puberty is influenced by genetic factors, nutrition, and general health. Delay in menarche has been reported in athletes, especially among those competing in leanness sports, and to be related to genetics and LEA.

Menstrual irregularity and menstrual dysfunction have for decades been associated with strenuous training, causing amenorrhea in athletes. However, today controlled studies have proven that a number of factors (including genetic factors, such as polycystic ovarian syndrome) can affect menstrual status. Furthermore, it is not strenuous training per se that causes menstrual dysfunction, but in some athletes, it is rather the relative energy deficiency. The latter factor may lead to hypo-estrogenism and negative consequences on bone strength, as described in this chapter. Therefore, to prevent menstrual dysfunction, female athletes, coaches, and medical personnel should learn how to optimize energy and nutrient intake and how nutrition and eating behavior relate to performance and health.

Effect of the menstrual cycle on performance

There is no conclusive evidence to suggest that menstrual function affects physical performance. With a few exceptions (for example, in women with serious dysmenorrhea), physical performance is not altered by the menstrual phase. Possibly, there is a phase of the cycle in which a particular athlete may be more or less efficient, but the difference is very small. At elite levels of performance, these slight variations may be of more significance. In situations where the athlete experiences impaired physical capacity due to menses, it is important that the athlete and the coach have a mutual understanding of how to optimize the training schedule to avoid negative consequences.

The pregnant athlete

Exercise of moderate intensity is safe during uncomplicated pregnancy. The American College of Obstetricians and Gynecologists and the ACSM state that a woman with a low-risk pregnancy can continue an already-established exercise regimen (for more than 30 minutes per day) or begin a new exercise program. Furthermore, research shows that combining regular exercise and pregnancy appears to benefit both mother and baby in many ways. More vigorous exercise is also regarded as safe for women who are well trained before the pregnancy. However, female athletes and physicians are concerned that regular maternal training during pregnancy may cause miscarriage, premature delivery, poor fetal growth, or musculoskeletal injury. For normal pregnancies, these concerns have not been substantiated.

A more controversial issue has been intensive training during pregnancy. The competing female athlete tends to maintain a more strenuous training schedule throughout pregnancy and resumes high-intensity postpartum training sooner. The concerns of pregnant competitive athletes fall into two general categories: (i) the effects of pregnancy on competitive ability, and (ii) the effects of strenuous training and competition on pregnancy and the fetus. Such athletes may require close obstetric supervision.

Some elite athletes plan to deliver a baby in between competitions such as the Olympic Games or World Championships. They want to maintain a high level of performance throughout pregnancy. Most studies show a small or moderate increase of the baseline in fetal heart rate (FHR) during or after maternal exercise. FHR deacceleration and bradycardia are uncommon. A common and simple way to monitor training intensity is to record maternal heart rate (MHR) during exercise. Target MHR zones and guidelines for exercise during pregnancy have been published, but these guidelines are developed for moderately exercising pregnant women only. The critical issue of volume blood flow to the pregnant uterus during exercise has been sparsely studied.

A recent Norwegian study examined the effects of strenuous treadmill running. Fetal well-being and utero placental blood flow were tested during strenuous treadmill running in the second trimester. The elite endurance-trained athletes were tested once at 23–29 weeks of pregnancy. Results showed that mean uterine artery volume blood flow was reduced to 60–80% after warming up and stayed at 40–75% of the initial value during exercise. FHR was within the normal range (110–160 bpm) as long as the woman exercised below 90% of maximal MHR. FHR normalized quickly after stopping the exercise. Thus, in this study on highly endurance-trained athletes, it was concluded that exercise at intensity above 90% of maximal MHR in pregnant elite athletes may compromise fetal well-being. This study was not designed to assess long-term outcomes after intensive training during pregnancy.

Further research on endurance-trained pregnant athletes is needed due to the fact that the number of female athletes who want to combine an athletic career with having family and children is increasing, since the average age of competitive female endurance athletes seems to be increasing. A limitation of these studies is the small sample size. The number of eligible women was limited because only pregnant Olympic-level athletes in endurance events were included. Therefore, it cannot be stated whether the results can be generalized to other groups of women who may be less physically fit but train regularly.

Postpartum

Many of the physiologic and morphologic changes of pregnancy persist 4–6 weeks postpartum. Thus, pregnancy exercise routines may be resumed gradually as soon as it is physically and medically safe. This will vary from one individual to another, with some women able to resume an exercise routine within days of delivery. There are no published studies to indicate that, in the absence of medical complications, rapid resumption of activities will result in adverse effects.

From practical experience with elite endurance-trained athletes, it should be emphasized that during the postpartum period, with its combination of resumption of training and breastfeeding, the mother should be encouraged to prepare for adequate recovery time and procedures – specifically, enough sleep, energy, and fluid intake.

The male paddler

Sprint canoe and kayak racing has been included in the Olympic Games since 1936, and while there were initially 10 000 m events, since 1960 the racing has been over 500 and 1000 m distances for men and only 500 m for women. Slalom was introduced at the 1972 Games and then returned on a regular basis in 1996. The physical and anthropometric characteristics of elite slalom and sprint competitors vary considerably. An examination of photographs from the 1936 Games in comparison to current athletes will demonstrate changes in size and muscle definition; however, there are no optimal physical size and proportionality characteristics of world-class paddlers. This serves to emphasize the comprehensive interaction of the many factors that lead to success in canoe sport.

At the 2012 Games in London, 200 m events were added for men's single canoe, men's single and double kayak, and women's single kayak. This separated the energy systems used in high-performance sport even more; the aerobic contributions for the 1000, 500, and 200 m have been estimated

at 82, 62, and 37%, respectively. Anaerobic capacity alone can predict performance in the 200 m events, and the sport has been changed significantly. Traditionally, athletes would compete at both 500 and 1000 m distances, but the introduction of the 200 m distance has resulted in specialized training for performances that are less than 40 seconds. These athletes have shorter but more intense training sessions, and resistance exercise plays a larger role in their preparation. Van Someren has reported that an increase of 1% in hull friction drag results in a reduction of boat speed of 0.27%. However, an increase in power output of 1% will increase boat speed by 0.33%. Thus, athletes can afford to increase body dimensions and absolute physiological capacities in order to improve performance. Although there are very little data on the anthropometric and physiological characteristics of the athletes who compete at this distance, international-level athletes are reported to have greater chest, upper-arm, and forearm circumferences; bi-epicondylar humeral breadth; and estimates of mesomorphy. Whether this is through training or natural selection is unknown.

There is literature describing the anthropometric features of international sprint canoe and kayak athletes competing in the 500 and 1000 m events. Significant differences exist in height, body mass, sitting height, and upper-extremity and forearm circumferences between international- versus national-level competitors in the 500 and 1000 m events. Medalists tend to be slightly larger in height and weight in comparison to their less successful peers, and comparative data between Olympics have demonstrated an increase in body mass, likely due to the specificity of training necessary for Olympic competition.

The proportionality profiles for both genders of paddlers are similar (Figure 3.1).

It is evident that they both have greater than average shoulder and chest breadths, large upper-body girths, low skinfold totals, greater than average proportional thigh lengths, and narrow hips in the male paddlers. There are surprisingly little peer-reviewed data on slalom paddlers.

Recent work has suggested that factors associated with the ACTN3XX genotype in male canoe and

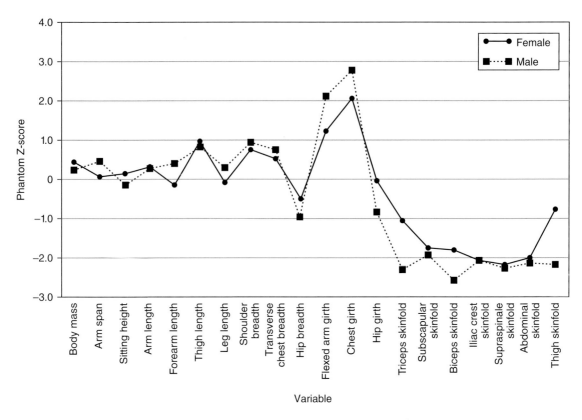

Figure 3.1 Relative body size of male and female Olympic sprint paddlers. *Source*: Ackland et al. (2003). Reproduced with permission of Elsevier.

kayak paddlers may provide a competitive advantage in the 1000 m event, but not the 200 m. The door to genomics in competitive canoeing has been opened.

Bibliography

Ackland, T.R., Ong, K.B., Kerr, D.A., and Ridge, B. (2003). Morphological characteristics of Olympic sprint canoe and kayak paddlers. *J Sci Med Sport* 6: 285–294.

Bishop, D. (2000). Physiological predictors of flat-water kayak performance in women. *Eur J Appl Physiol* 82: 91–97.

Michael, J.S., Rooney, K.B., and Smith, R. (2008). The metabolic demands of kayaking: a review. *J Sports Sci Med* 7: 1–7.

Mountjoy, M., Sundgot-Borgen, J., Burke, L. et al. (2014). The IOC consensus statement: beyond the female athlete triad—relative energy deficiency in sport (RED-S). *Br J Sports Med* 48: 491–497.

Sundgot-Borgen, J. and Garthe, I. (2011). Elite athletes in aesthetic and Olympic weight-class sports and the challenge of body weight and body compositions. *J Sports Sci* 29 (Suppl 1): S101–S114.

Sundgot-Borgen, J., Meyer, N.L., Loham, T.G. et al. (2013). How to minimize the health risks to athletes who compete in weight-sensitive sports review and position statement on behalf of the Ad Hoc Research Working Group on Body Composition, Health and Performance, under the auspices of the IOC Medical Commission. *Br J Sports Med* 47 (16): 1012–1022.

van Someren, K.A. and Howatson, G. (2013). Prediction of flatware kayaking performance. *Int J Sports Physiol Perform* 3: 207–218.

Chapter 4
Physiology of canoeing

Hans Rosdahl[1], Jose Calbet[2,3], A. William Sheel[4], and Robert Boushel[4]

[1]Swedish School of Sport and Health Sciences, Stockholm, Sweden

[2]Department of Physical Education, University of Las Palmas de Gran Canaria, Las Palmas de Gran Canaria, Spain

[3]Research Institute of Biomedical and Health Sciences (IUIBS), University of Las Palmas de Gran Canaria, Las Palmas de Gran Canaria, Spain

[4]School of Kinesiology, Faculties of Education and Medicine, The University of British Columbia, Vancouver, BC, Canada

Introduction

Advances in the field of physiology have led to new approaches to study diverse physiological components of athletic performance ranging from the molecular level to integrative systemic responses. Knowledge of the physiology of elite canoeing performance has gradually increased over the last decade, while new avenues of research on the physiology of athletic performance and the physiological responses to training are being applied across a wide range of sports. In addition, there is an increasing integration of knowledge from different disciplines within physiology (neurophysiology, metabolism) and between different fields (e.g., biomechanics, nutrition, and biochemistry) that opens new possibilities to enrich our understanding of performance factors in canoeing that also can be applied to training approaches for athletes. The aim of this review is to build upon previous comprehensive reviews on canoeing and provide a basis for future directions in research in the physiology of the sport.

World best performance times

The world best times of the winners at the different racing distances are summarized in Table 4.1 as a general base to understand the physiological and energy demands in the canoe sprint discipline. The race times included are taken from tables published by the International Canoe Federation (ICF). These include the world best times of winners during official races in the finals of the ICF events from 1975 to 2013. Official ICF events are Olympic Games, World Championships, European Championships, World Cups, Continental Championships, and other canoe sprint events. As evident, there is a large span ranging from about 30 seconds to about 20 minutes in the racing times between the shortest and longest distances. This unquestionably entails physiological and training consequences. Interestingly, the time differences between men and women appear consistent (11–15%) for each distance across single kayak, double kayak, or four-person kayak (K1, K2, or K4, respectively) for kayak competitions. Additionally, the summary shows very similar world best times for female kayakers versus male canoeists with all crews (K1, K2, or K4). Figure 4.1 shows the number of best times for winners from 1992 to 2013. Notably, most of the best times were attained over the last 10 years studied (i.e. from 2003 to 2013).

Bioenergetic contributions to different racing distances

Peak paddling performance depends upon maximal metabolic power (aerobic and anaerobic) complemented with superior locomotion economy.

Canoeing, First Edition. Edited by Don McKenzie and Bo Berglund.
© 2019 International Olympic Committee. Published 2019 by John Wiley & Sons Ltd.

Table 4.1 World best times of winners until 2013 from ICF world top athletes list in canoe sprint.

	Kayaking – men						
	200 m		**500 m**		**1000 m**		**5000 m**
	Time (s)	*Time (s)*	Time (min·s)	*Time (s)*	Time (min·s)	*Time (s)*	
K1	33.980	*33.98*	1.35630	*95.63*	3.22485	*202.49*	18.00040
K2	31.182	*31.18*	1.26873	*86.87*	3.07095	*186.87*	
K3	29.023	*29.02*	1.19650	*79.65*	2.47734	*167.74*	
	Kayaking – women						
	200 m		**500 m**		**1000 m**		**5000 m**
	Time (s)	*Time (s)*	Time (min·s)	*Time (s)*	Time (min·s)	*Time (s)*	
K1	38.970	*38.97*	1.47066	107.07	3.52461	232.46	20.10100
K2	35.878	*35.88*	1.37071	97.07	3.31741	211.74	
K3	33.778	*33.78*	1.30719	90.72	3.13296	193.30	
	Time differences Kayak women vs kayak men (s)						
	200 m	**500 m**	**1000 m**				
K1	5.0	11.4	30.0				
K2	4.7	10.2	24.9				
K3	4.8	11.1	25.6				
	Canoeing – men						
	200 m		**500 m**		**1000 m**		**5000 m**
	Time (s)	*Time (s)*	Time (min·s)	*Time (s)*	Time (min·s)	*Time (s)*	
C1	38.383	*38.380*	1.45614	*105.61*	3.46201	*226.2*	20.27350
C2	35.760	*35.800*	1.38020	*98.02*	3.28531	*208.53*	
C3	32.753	*32.750*	1.29956	*89.96*	3.14459	*194.46*	
	Time differences: kayak women vs. canoeing men (s)						
	200 m	**500 m**	**1000 m**				
K1	−0.6	−1.5	−6.3				
K2	−0.1	−0.9	−3.2				
K3	−1.0	−0.8	−1.2				
	Canoeing – women						
	200 m	**500 m**					
C1	47.542	–					
C2	–	1.59976					

Elite canoeists have highly developed aerobic (oxidative phosphorylation) and anaerobic (phosphagen and glycolytic) capacities, and both systems are integrally involved in all canoeing events in a continuum with work (power × time) demand. The relative contribution of each energy system thus depends on the distance of the event, with the short distances relying more heavily on anaerobic power, progressing to increased reliance on aerobic power with increasing distance and duration of the event (Figure 4.2). The range of competition distances from 200 to 10000 m implies quite different metabolic profiles of sprint athletes compared to the distance competitor. The short-distance events require the canoeist to generate explosive power, as seen by the world records for men and women ranging from approximately 30 seconds for 200 m, to approximately 1:35 for 500 m and 3.5–4 minutes

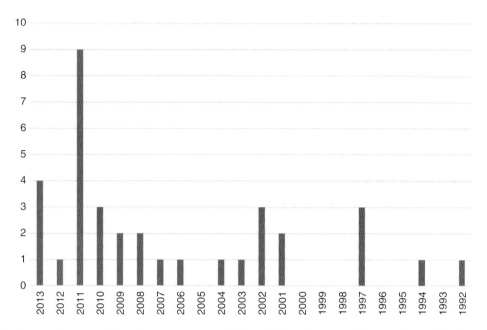

Figure 4.1 The number of best times for winners from 1992 to 2013 in ICF events (Olympic Games, World Championships, European Championships, World Cups, Continental Championships, and other canoe sprint events). Most of the best times were attained over the last 10 years that were studied.

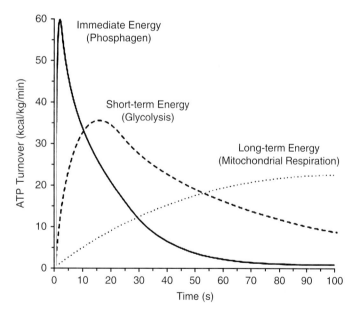

Figure 4.2 Contribution of skeletal muscle energy systems to total energy output during exercise. The relative contribution of each energy system depends on the distance of the event, with the short distances relying more heavily on anaerobic power, progressing to increased reliance on aerobic power with increasing distance and duration of the event.

for 1000 m (Table 4.1, "World best times"), while the 10000 m event lasts for 45 minutes and demands high aerobic power. For the 100 and 200 m events, a highly developed muscle mass is required to generate large forces to accelerate the

canoe to top speed, and in the initial seconds energy is provided by stored adenosine triphosphate (ATP), phosphocreatine (PCr) breakdown, and glycolysis. In a sprint lasting 6 seconds, about 50% of the energy is provided by the glycolytic metabolism. The arms rely even more on the glycolytic metabolism than the legs, and this is especially so in canoeing. Canoeists can reach peak power outputs of >1100W over 10 seconds, and can sustain 360–400W over a 1 minute time trial. High creatine–phosphate stores are critical for sprint events and can be depleted rapidly within 30 seconds. As can be seen from Figure 4.2, the contribution of the energy systems is a function of time and ATP demand. At the onset of exercise, stored high-energy phosphates are utilized first, followed by glycolysis and oxidative pathways. Maximal glycolytic rate in muscle is reached within approximately 10 seconds but can be even shorter (~6 seconds), and in a 100 m canoe event, peak blood lactate levels can be in excess of 20 mM measured after the event. If a sprint is performed at the end of a race competition (final sprint), there will be an important contribution of anaerobic metabolism.

The aerobic contribution to different paddling distances is determined by measuring oxygen uptake in both laboratory simulations and on water, while the anaerobic component has been estimated by the use of the accumulated oxygen deficit (AOD). Data from a limited number of studies in kayaking are shown in Table 4.2. For the 200 m distance, current data indicate approximately 40% aerobic and 60% anaerobic contribution. The actual anaerobic contribution is likely a bit higher because stored O_2 (myoglobin, etc.) cannot be computed with the AOD method. The aerobic contribution for the 1000 m is in the range of 80–86 and 60–69% for the 500 m distance. There are insufficient data available comparing men and women; however, the estimated aerobic energy contributions are thought to be similar.

Maximal aerobic power of kayakers and canoeists

Maximal aerobic power is synonymous with maximal oxygen uptake (VO_2 max), which is the maximal volume of oxygen that an individual can take up and utilize during exhaustive exercise using large muscle groups. A high VO_2 max appears a requisite trait of elite paddlers. Dating back to the first measurements in the 1960s, it has been known that competitive paddlers have a high VO_2 max. Elite national-level male kayakers have VO_2 max values of approximately 70 ml·kg^{-1}·min^{-1} measured on a kayak ergometer (see Table 4.1). Recordings of VO_2 max on the water (kayaking or canoeing) are limited, but across a number of studies, values in the range of 59–69 ml·kg^{-1}·min^{-1} have been reported. In women, VO_2 max is lower, in the range of 53–59 ml·kg^{-1}·min^{-1}. Since most investigations have been carried out with mixed groups of kayakers and canoeists (i.e. not homogeneous groups and not specific to the racing distances' specialties), the precise VO_2 max levels required for top performances at the different racing distances remain to be investigated more carefully. In addition, supplementary data are required on the physical characteristics of elite female and male canoeists. Most of the VO_2 max values reported between 1960 and 2015 are listed in Tables 4.3 and 4.4 to assist the reader with an overview of the available data on VO_2 max of male and female kayakers and canoeists measured during either treadmill running, ergometer cycling, kayaking on water, or kayak ergometry. The tables are constructed to include both the historical progress and the most important methodological aspects that the reader can consider in assessing the results.

Methodological aspects of maximal aerobic power

The main criterion generally used to define that VO_2 max has been attained during a single test is no further increase in oxygen uptake despite an increase in exercise intensity (i.e. a "leveling off" or plateau in VO_2). Frequently used supplemental criteria are a respiratory exchange ratio larger than 1.1–1.15, and a blood lactate concentration above 8–9 mmol·l^{-1} measured 5 minutes after the end of exercise. However, these criteria were developed for whole-body exercise conditions, meaning that at least the muscle mass of both lower extremities was involved in the exercise.

Table 4.2 Aerobic and anaerobic energy contributions at different canoeing racing distances.

Reference	Methodological notes		Participants	200 m			500 m			1000 m		
				Aerobic (%)	Anaerobic (%)	Time (sec)	Aerobic (%)	Anaerobic (%)	Time (sec)	Aerobic (%)	Anaerobic (%)	Time (sec)
Zouhal et al. (2012)	Open water	AOD	French national level (n = 7 men)	–	–	–	78.3	21.7	108	86.6	13.4	224
Bishop (2000)	Ergometer	AOD	Australian national and international competitors (n = 9 women)	–	–	–	70.3	29.8	120	–	–	–
Byrnes and Kearny (1997, abstr.) and Kearny and McKenzie (2000)	Ergometer	Average VO$_2$	USA national team, 1996 (n = 10; 6 men and 4 women)	36.5	63	–	63.5	38	–	84.5	18	–
Byrnes and Kearny (1997, abstr.) and Kearny and McKenzie (2000)	Ergometer	Average VO$_2$	USA national team, 1996 (n = 6 men)	37.8	–	–	62.8	–	–	82.2	–	–
Byrnes and Kearny (1997, abstr.) and Kearny and McKenzie (2000)	Ergometer	Average VO$_2$	USA national team, 1996 (n = 4 women)	40	–	–	69	–	–	86	–	–
Zamparo et al. (1999)	Open water	–	Italian middle-high class athletes (n = 8; 3 men and 5 women)	*250 m* 40.5	59.4	–	60.4	40.3	–	83.3	16.7	–
Fernandez et al. (1995, abstr.)	Ergometer	AOD	World Championship finalists (n = 9)	43.5	56.5	56.8	62.9	37.1	124	79.7	20.3	255

Table 4.3 VO₂ max for kayakers and canoeists reported in the literature between 1960 and 2015.

Men

Reference	Participants	Age (years)	BM (kg)	Mode	VO₂ max ($l\,min^{-1}$)	VO₂ max ($ml \times kg^{-1} \times min^{-1}$)	Best performance times (s) 500 m	1000 m	200 m
Lundgren et al. (2015)	Norway elite kayakers (n = 11 men)	19.6	78.4	Treadmill	5.78±0.56	73.7±6.3			
Borges et al. (2012)	Portugal elite kayak paddlers (n = 8 men)	22±4.2	77.2±6.7	Treadmill?	4.72	61.2±5.5			
Misigoj-Durakovic and Heimer (1992)	Croatia (n =18, a group of kayakers being candidates for the 1987 Universiade)	–	75.1±6.4	Treadmill	4.6±0.57	63±7.2			
Tesch (1983)	Sweden (n = 6; national caliber, incl. five on the Olympic team)	22±3	80±6	Treadmill	5.36 (range 5.11–5.66)	67			
Thomson and Scrutton (1978)	Canada (n = 4, national competitors in Canada)	19	75.3±6.3	Treadmill	4.6±0.5	60.6±4.6			
Tesch (1976)	Sweden (n = 4 elite competitors of European and World Championships and Olympic Games, 1952–1972)	25 (22–28)	78 (73–81)	Treadmill	5.4 (range 4.7–6.1)	69.2			
Gollnick et al. (1972)	Sweden (n = 4 elite, including an Olympic and World Champion)	26 (25–27)	74 (71–79)	Bicycle ergometer/ Treadmill	4.2	56.8 (55–58)			
Saltin and Åstrand (1967)	Sweden (n = 4 national team, 1963–1964)	–	–	Arm and leg exercise	5.1	70			
Saltin (1967)	Sweden (n = 1, Olympic Champion in kayaking 1964)	23	72	Bicycle ergometer	4.52	62.8			
Zouhal et al. (2012)	France national level (n = 7 men)	21.9±1.7	78.5±3.4	Kayaking *on water*	5.34	68.8±8	102±1	216±2	
Gomes et al. (2012)	Portugal elite (n = 6 men)	24.2±4.8	79.7±8.5	Kayak ergometer	5.36±0.58	68.1±6.2			
Buglione et al. (2011)	Italy kayak teams (n = 46 men)	17.9±2.7	78.2±6.1	Kayaking **on water**	4.79±0.35	61.4±4.4			
Garcia Pallares et al. (2010a)	Spain elite (n = 10, incl. two Olympic gold medalists)	25.6±2.5	85.2±4.6	Kayak ergometer	5.80	68.1±3.1			
Garcia-Pallares et al. (2010b)	Spain elite (n = 14, incl. two Olympic gold medalists)	25.2±2.5	84.9	Kayak ergometer	5.84	68.8			
Michael et al. (2010)	Australia elite (n = 10: 5 international experience, 5 national)	25±6	84.9±5.8	Kayak ergometer	4.66±0.28	54.9			
Garcia-Pallares et al. (2009)	Spain elite (n = 11, incl. two Olympic gold medalists)	26.2±2.8	86.2±5.2	Kayak ergometer	5.87	68.1			
van Someren and Howatson (2008)	Great Britain (n = 18: 10 international experience, 8 club level)	25±4	83.2±5.2	Kayak ergometer	4.55±0.46	54.7	122.1±5.7	262.6±36.4	41.6±2.1
Forbes and Chilibeck (2007)	Canadian (n = 10, recruited from local club with a range in experience)	19.9±2.3	76.3±10.6	Kayak ergometer	3.64±0.43	48±4.0			

Table 4.4 VO$_2$ max for kayakers and canoeists reported in the literature between 1960 and 2015.

Reference	Participants	Age (years)	BM (kg)	Mode	VO$_2$ max (l min^{-1})	VO$_2$ max (ml × kg^{-1} × min^{-1})	Best performance times (s) 500 m	Best performance times (s) 1000 m	Best performance times (s) 200 m
Men									
van Someren and Palmer (2003)	Great Britain (n = 13, 200 m international racing experience)	26±5	84.5±4.9	Kayak ergometer	4.45±0.55	52.6±4.9			39.9±0.8
van Someren and Palmer (2003)	Great Britain (n = 13, 200 m national racing experience)	25±6	79.9±7.8	Kayak ergometer	4.25±0.35	54.5±5.6			42.6±0.9
van Someren et al. (2000)	Great Britain (n = 9, high club level to national squad level)	24±4	77.3±6.4	Kayak ergometer	4.27±0.58	55.2			
Fry and Morton (1991)	Australia (n = 7, selected state representatives)	26.1±7.3	81.05±10.26	Kayak ergometer	4.78±0.60	59.22±7.1	121.7±10.0	249.1±19.3	
Fry and Morton (1991)	Australia (n = 31, nonselected state representatives)	25.4±7.4	70.66±7.99	Kayak ergometer	3.87±0.75	54.80±8.4	140.6±13.1	280.1±27.7	
Tesch (1983)	Sweden (n = 6 national caliber, incl. five on the Olympic team)	22±3	80±6	Kayaking on water	4.67 (range, 4.48–4.87)	58.4			
Thomson and Scrutton (1978)	Canada (n = 4, national competitors in Canada)	19	75.3±6.3	Kayak ergometer	3.4±0.6	45.4±6.6			
Tesch (1976)	Sweden (n = 4 elite competitors of European and World Championships and Olympic Games 1952–1972)	25 (22–28)	78 (73–81)	Kayaking on water	4.7 (range 4.6–5.0)	57.7			
Gollnick et al. (1972)	Sweden (n = 4 elite, including an Olympic and World Champion)	26 (25–27)	74 (71–79)	Arm cranking	4.06	54.9 (51–60)			
Saltin (1967)	Sweden (n = 1, Olympic Champion in kayaking 1964)	23	72	Kayaking on water	4.27	59.3			
Women									
Gomes et al. (2012)	Portugal elite kayak paddlers (n = 6 women)	24.3±4.5	65.4±3.5	Kayak ergometer	3.83±0.35	58.5±5.59			
Buglione et al. (2011)	Italy kayak teams (n = 23 women)	17.8±2.5	66.0±6.6	Kayaking on water	3.46±0.31	52.6±4.3			
Forbes and Chilibeck (2007)	Canada (n = 5, recruited from local club with a range in experience)	18.2±2.4	61.6±5.2	Kayak ergometer	2.86±0.23	46.6±4.0			
Bishop (2000)	Australia (n = 9, range from international to national level)	23±5	70.4±6.3	Kayak ergometer	3.00±0.30	44.81±6.02			
Male Canoeists									
Buglione et al. (2011)	Italy kayak teams (n = 5 men)	17.9±2.7	76.8±3.5	Canoeing on water	4.75±0.45	61.8±4.0			
Misigoj-Durakovic and Heimer (1992)	Croatia? (n = 11, a group of canoeists being candidates for the 1987 Universiade)	–	80.2±9.0	Treadmill	4.9±0.58	61.6±4.4			

Several other methodological aspects are essential to consider when evaluating individual VO_2 max data of kayakers, when analyzing data between different laboratories, and when comparing VO_2 max between different sports. It is, for instance, fundamental to have information accessible on the validity and reliability of the equipment used for the VO_2 determination. The Douglas Bag method is still considered the most valid and reliable method for both laboratory and field conditions (i.e. the golden standard, provided it is correctly handled). Fortunately, the Douglas Bag method was used in the first investigations of kayakers in the mid-1960s and in some subsequent studies during the 1970s and 1980s (Tables 4.3 and 4.4). However, in recent years, automated metabolic systems have been used by many investigators in spite of convincing evidence they need careful evaluation. Hence, to obtain comparable data, it would be necessary that each investigator demonstrate how well their measurement system agrees with the Douglas Bag method and likewise to demonstrate high precision (i.e. coefficient of variation [CV] less than 2%) when measuring elite kayakers with automated systems. Moreover, the type of exercise and muscle recruitment is crucial to consider since the mechanisms limiting VO_2 max are different when using large and small muscle groups. VO_2 max for kayakers has been reported during treadmill running, ergometer cycling, arm cranking, kayak ergometry, and kayaking on water. A majority of the data in the literature have, however, been collected during kayak ergometry, likely because this entails acceptable specificity and validity. Another consideration is whether the measurements have been performed during the racing season or off-season.

It has been suggested that performance is better indicated if the maximal aerobic power of kayakers is expressed in absolute terms (VO_2 l·min^{-1}) compared to that relative to body mass (VO_2 ml·kg^{-1}·min^{-1}). The rationale for this is that the body mass is supported by the kayak and that a few extra kilos result in insignificantly higher resistance. This proposal was made when the roles concerning the dimensions of the kayak were stricter and did not allow any kayaks being adapted to the kayaker's body mass as they are currently.

Consequently, there is a need to further investigate whether it is most appropriate to express the aerobic power of kayakers in absolute or relative terms and to determine potential differences between the racing distances.

Determinants of aerobic capacity

Aerobic capacity can be defined as the highest rate of VO_2 that can be sustained during exercise. Thus, the aerobic energy production depends on the absolute VO_2 max and the percentage of VO_2 max that can be sustained throughout the event. The VO_2 max levels of elite canoeists (60–70 ml·min^{-1}·kg^{-1}) are generally lower than those for elite skiers, cyclists, and runners (up to ~90 ml·min^{-1}·kg^{-1}), and this has been thought to relate to the fact that while canoeists have a highly developed musculature in the torso, less total muscle mass is engaged, or activated intensively relative to total body mass. The fact that well-trained paddlers can achieve 80–85% of their arm + leg or treadmill VO_2 max during arm cranking alone indicates highly refined oxygen transport and utilization systems. As athletes have applied more sophisticated training approaches in recent years and body dimensions have also become more refined, the question of optimal muscle mass needs re-examination.

The underlying physiological components of VO_2 max are the capacity of the circulation to deliver oxygen and the extraction rate of O_2 by muscles. It is well-known that in trained athletes performing whole-body exercise, the dominant factor in the equation is O_2 delivery, and accordingly maximal cardiac output and muscle blood flow. During arm exercise, peak VO_2 values are achieved at lower cardiac output values than during whole-body exercise in physically active subjects. Nevertheless, the work performed by the heart is greater at near-exhaustion during incremental arm-cranking exercise than leg pedaling, indicating that the pumping capacity of the heart or the maximal cardiac output is a key determining factor in canoeing endurance performance.

Pulmonary ventilation

During heavy exercise, there is a significant increase in muscle metabolism, with corresponding decreases in mixed venous O_2 content and increases in mixed venous CO_2 pressure (PCO_2) to exceed 80 mmHg. As such, there is an increased demand for alveolar-to-arterial gas exchange. However, with intense exercise, the high cardiac output means that blood spends less time in the pulmonary capillaries to accomplish this exchange. The healthy pulmonary system, as the body's first and last lines of defense for O_2 and CO_2 transport, generally meets these challenges with an appropriate increase in alveolar ventilation such that alveolar PO_2 and PCO_2 are well regulated. The respiratory musculature (both inspiratory and expiratory muscles) is equally well suited to meet the ventilatory demands of exercise and is capable of sustaining prolonged force development for the generation of airflow. The ventilatory response to kayaking and canoeing may differ from that for other "aerobic" activities such as running, cycling, and cross-country skiing in at least two ways:

Upper limb. Exercise performed with the upper body elicits distinct metabolic and cardiorespiratory responses compared to lower-body exercise. For example, with arm exercise, there are lower maximal values for ventilation, heart rate, and O_2 uptake. It is generally agreed upon that the differences relate to the smaller muscle mass involved with upper-limb exercise. For a given level of submaximal power output, upper-limb exercise is associated with higher ventilation relative to lower-body exercise.

Entrainment. There are medullary neural networks and sensory reflex mechanisms that control breathing such that there is precise regulation of breathing pattern and breath duty cycle. For the most part, the respiratory system (control system, respiratory musculature, and airways) is able to meet the demands of heavy exercise where arterial blood gases are maintained at near-resting levels. During kayaking and canoeing, ventilation is coupled or "entrained" with locomotion where the stroke rate can be coupled to the breathing rate. For example, elite kayakers who involuntarily select a breathing frequency-to-stroke rate of 1:1 had consistently lower oxyhemoglobin saturation values at peak exercise than those who selected a 1:2 ratio. It is possible that entrainment may pose a mechanical restraint on the ventilatory response during canoeing, but this requires further study.

The circulation

Maximal cardiac output and the distribution of blood flow to the limbs and trunk have not been measured in elite canoeists, but comparisons can be made to other sports. In cyclists, rowers, and skiers, maximal cardiac outputs in excess of $35 l \cdot min^{-1}$ have been recorded, and blood flow to the legs measured by thermodilution is between 24 and $30 l \cdot min^{-1}$, representing up to 85% of the cardiac output. The trunk and brain receive an estimated $4-5 l \cdot min^{-1}$. Based on the maximal VO_2 values in canoeists, it is estimated that their cardiac outputs are in the range of $25-30 l \cdot min^{-1}$, depending on body size. In canoeing, the legs are significantly engaged in the paddle stroke and therefore also receive a significant portion of the cardiac output, but likely lower than in rowing. Nonetheless, a physiological challenge in canoeing is that a finite cardiac output must be shared between the upper body and legs. In elite cross-country skiers with a maximal cardiac output of approximately $31 l \cdot min^{-1}$, the legs receive blood flows of $18 l \cdot min^{-1}$ and the arms approximately $8-9 l \cdot min^{-1}$. As a closer comparison to canoeing, during two-arm cranking on an ergometer, the legs receive approximately 30% of the cardiac output ($\sim 6-8 l \cdot min^{-1}$) despite the fact that the legs act more as stabilizing muscles for arm and torso work, as in canoeing. When both arms and legs are dynamically engaged simultaneously, the amount of blood perfusing each extremity depends on the adjustments of the regional conductances (flow/mean arterial pressure), which is dictated by the exercise mode, as shown by invasive procedures in cross-country skiers and physically active subjects. For example, during incremental double-poling exercise in cross-country skiers, the perfusion of the arms is higher than during skiing with the diagonal technique (i.e. when the main propulsive muscles are in the legs).

To achieve the high perfusion in the arms required during canoeing, blood flow to the legs must be restricted by sympathetic vasoconstriction due to the fact that the peak cardiac output cannot maximally perfuse both the arm and leg muscles simultaneously and at the same time maintain the arterial blood pressure. It is known that training induces alteration of the distribution of flow to the most activated muscle groups, and this is mediated by an interplay between local vasodilatory mechanisms and the sympathetic nervous system. This is exemplified by the finding that oxygen uptake of the arms is elevated after ski training by redistribution of a greater proportion of the cardiac output to the arms compared to the legs, mediated by sympathetic vasoconstriction in the legs without change in peak cardiac output. The larger proportion of blood flow to the arms occurs despite that the percentage of type I fibers and capillary density per unit mass are significantly lower in the arms (deltoids and triceps) compared to the legs (quadriceps). Detailed studies on the specific regional hemodynamic patterns in canoeists are an important area of future research and are awaited with interest.

High cardiac outputs in endurance athletes are characterized by a large stroke volume that depends on cardiac chamber size, cardiac chamber mechanics, and ventricular performance. Endurance athletes have a markedly greater ability to use the Starling mechanism to increase stroke volume. This is primarily due to a large end-diastolic volume, which has been measured as high as 250 ml. Large end-diastolic volumes are endowed characteristics, but years of training are likely to enhance chamber size due to greater cardiac chamber compliance, and also a very rapid diastolic relaxation time, which actually generates diastolic suction from the left atrium across the mitral valve into the apex of the left ventricle. Similarly, the longitudinal axis shortening of the heart is a key feature of the maximal pumping capacity of the heart, as seen in athletes who have trained for many years. The high VO_2 max values reported in top kayakers imply a high cardiac output, greater perfusion of the arm muscles, and hence different hemodynamic adjustments. While during leg exercise the afterload of the heart (as indicated by the greater mean arterial pressure) increases moderately, it does to a greater extent during arm exercise. This allows for an increase in the perfusion of the arm muscles by increasing the perfusion pressure. This has a price, however, as a high afterload during arm exercise may limit the peak pumping capacity of the heart. In elite kayakers, regular training with high afterload is the most plausible mechanism for the observed heart adaptations of a remarkably high ventricular mass with chamber dimensions similar to those observed in healthy sedentary men. More studies are required to understand what factors limit cardiac output in canoeists and how cardiac output is distributed during training and peak performance power output.

Primary muscles and fiber characteristics

From electromyography (EMG) analysis, the anterior deltoid is the most activated muscle group throughout the stroke. The trapezius, triceps, and rectus abdominus are engaged at a lower level of activation, while the biceps, latissimus dorsi, and pectoralis major are activated for approximately 20% of the stroke. The lower body plays a central role in stabilizing the torso but has a limited range of motion during muscle contraction. These muscle groups include the hip flexors, knee extensors, and ankle extensors. As muscle power is essential in canoeing, a relatively high proportion of type II myosin heavy-chain isoforms is an important attribute, with the ability to rapidly hydrolyze ATP and achieve rapid cross-bridge cycling and high ATP turnover rates. Fiber types have been determined in canoeists from biopsies of the gastrocnemius, vastus lateralis, deltoid, triceps, biceps brachii, and latissumus dorsi using primarily the ATPase staining method. Relatively high percentages of type II fibers (FT) have been found in the biceps (56% IIa; 14% IIx fibers), vastus (57% IIa; 17% IIx fibers), and lattisimus dorsi (56% IIa fibers). The cross-sectional area of muscle fibers of the arms is increased in canoeists with fiber areas that are larger in arm muscles than in leg muscles. Type II fibers generally show greater hypertrophy than type I (although this is not a fixed pattern), with fiber area ratios of 1.4 for type II/type I in the biceps compared to 1.1 in the vastus, reflecting accentuated loading patterns in the arms.

Mitochondrial volume in highly trained endurance athletes averages 8–9% of muscle volume in both arms and legs, which is more than twofold higher than in untrained individuals. Despite the general conception that type I fibers possess the highest mitochondrial volume and thus the highest aerobic potential, recent findings indicate that trained type IIa fibers contain similar volume density of mitochondria. The canoeist endowed with a high proportion of type IIa fibers thus has the advantage of a higher power output of muscle and a high ability to supply that power with aerobic pathways. Mitochondrial capacity to consume oxygen is in excess of the maximum oxygen that can be delivered by the circulation and therefore does not pose a limitation to VO_2 max. A main effect of a very high mitochondrial volume in skeletal muscle is that less lactate is formed at a given exercise load. A given energy demand requires a lower total oxidative phosphorylation rate per mitochondrial unit (i.e. less ATP production per unit mitochondria). The product of a lower unit ATP production demand for contractile activity yields a lower concentration of adenosine diphosphate (ADP), adenosine monophosphate, and Pi, and the result is less activation of glycogenolysis and glycolysis, and thus a lower lactate production.

The lower ATP production per unit mitochondria is not only a volume effect (more mitochondria) but also due to the fact that mitochondria are less sensitive to signal activation by ADP. Other regulatory changes in muscle mitochondria in highly trained athletes contribute to aerobic endurance performance. The capacity of mitochondria to oxidize fat is enhanced, and this occurs due to a larger volume of not only mitochondria but also per unit mitochondria. The precise mechanism for this latter effect is not known, but it is a clear advantage in sparing muscle glycogen and maintaining blood glucose for long-duration events. A larger mitochondrial volume is also linked to a higher affinity of mitochondria for oxygen. The effect on oxygen consumption is measurable in intact mitochondria defined by the mitochondrial p50, the PO_2 at which mitochondrial respiration is half-maximum.

A lower p50 indicates a higher affinity for O_2, and this can contribute to an increase in muscle VO_2 by decreasing mitochondrial PO_2 and increasing the diffusion gradient (Figure 4.3). This effect can account for approximately 100–200 ml higher VO_2 across the muscle with training and constitutes an important performance difference.

Elite endurance athletes are able to extract a high fraction of the arterial O_2 content, in the range of 85–90%, or approximately 10–20% higher than average individuals. This process can be measured by arteriovenous cannulation and reflects the component parameters of oxygen uptake (Figure 4.3) represented by Fick's law of diffusion: VO_2 max = O_2 diffusion capacity (DO_2) × (PO_2 capillary − PO_2 mitochondria); and the Fick principle: VO_2 max = O_2 delivery × arteriovenous O_2 difference). The primary factors underlying O_2 diffusion are the capillary density, the mean transit time of the erythrocytes, and the PO_2 gradient between capillary and mitochondria. The lower the mitochondrial PO_2, which is defined by the relative activation of mitochondria, the greater the O_2 gradient; and the higher the intensity of muscular work, the greater the activation of mitochondria and utilization of O_2. At peak exercise, mitochondrial PO_2 is very low (close to zero), creating a large pressure gradient from the capillary across the muscle. The absolute level of O_2 diffusion (ml·mmHg^{-1} pressure of O_2) is then largely defined by the capillary density, which both maximizes the contact points with the muscle membrane and also serves to slow the passage of red blood cells for offloading of O_2. Thus, elite canoeists must have a high capillary density in the upper body to maximize oxygen transfer to sustain muscular work. Capillary densities of 5–6 cap·mm² have been reported in endurance athletes and are generally similar in distribution in trained arms and legs despite a higher type I fiber type distribution in the legs (~60%) compared to arms (~40%). Despite this even distribution of capillaries, peak O_2 extraction rates are lower in the arms compared to legs. During incremental arm cranking, peak oxygen extractions are in the range of 70% in trained rowers. The lower extraction rates in the arms of trained rowers compared to those trained in leg cycling are due in part to a higher blood flow per unit mass in the

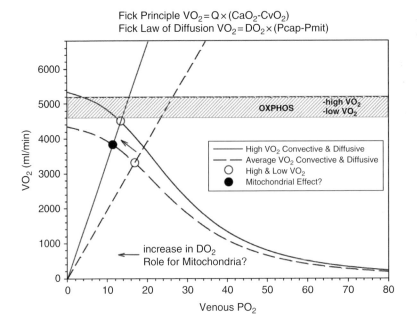

Figure 4.3 Model of convective and diffusive components of peak VO_2. Peak VO_2 during exercise represented by Fick's law of diffusion ($VO_2 = DO_2 \times [Pcap - Pmit]$) and the Fick principle ($VO_2 = Q \times [CaO_2 - CvO_2]$). The straight lines from the origin through the data points (circles) reflect Fick's law of diffusion (leg VO_2 per femoral venous PO_2). The sigmoid curves show the Fick principle defined as the product of blood flow and the arteriovenous O_2 difference (O_2 extraction). The higher sigmoid curve and left-shift of the straight line of $VO_2 - PvO_2$ shows a combined increase in blood flow and diffusion capacity to achieve a higher VO_2 max. The filled circle shows the theoretical increase in diffusion capacity for a given blood flow, owing to local muscle (mitochondria, capillaries) effects. The horizontal dashed region represents the numerical range of mitochondrial O_2 flux capacity, with different training status. CaO_2 = arterial $[O_2]$; cvO_2 = venous $[O_2]$; DO_2 = O_2 diffusion capacity; Pcap = mean capillary PO_2; Pmito = PO_2 at cytochrome c oxidase of mitochondria. The arrow shows a theoretical increase in DO_2 and VO_2 owing to regulatory changes in mitochondria.

arms and a reduced red blood cell transit time. In fact, the highest arm O_2 extraction values in cross-country skiers are observed during peak exercise with the classical diagonal technique (both arms and legs are contributing to the propulsive forces) when the arm blood flow is lower than during the double-poling technique (propulsive forces are predominantly generated by the arms) when the arm blood flow is much greater.

Lactate threshold and critical power

The exceptionally high metabolic requirements of elite-level canoeing necessitate a high maximal oxygen uptake, a high anaerobic capacity, muscle strength in the upper body, and technical efficiency. A major performance determinant in events lasting

longer than 1–2 minutes is a high peak VO_2 and a high fraction of the peak VO_2, which can be sustained before lactate progressively increases, or the lactate threshold. It has long been known that kayakers have high anaerobic thresholds or maximal sustainable lactate levels in the range of 80–85% of VO_2 max, and a similar pattern is presumed in canoeists. A significant correlation is between the lactate threshold and kayak performance at 200, 500, and 1000 m distances. Similar to the lactate threshold, critical power is the highest average work rate or power output that can be maintained over a specific period of time. It is mathematically defined as the power-asymptote of the hyperbolic relationship between power output and time-to-exhaustion. Physiologically, critical power represents the boundary between the steady-state and non-steady-state exercise intensity domains and therefore is a meaningful index of performance in addition to the lactate threshold and VO_2 max. Generally, time to exhaustion at the velocity of VO_2 max is inversely related to VO_2 max. The longer the canoeing event, the greater the reliance on aerobically generated ATP, but the absolute power output sustained by aerobic metabolism is significantly lower than the glycolytic system. In kayakers, VO_2 max velocity can be sustained for approximately 6 minutes. Any power output demand by muscle above that which can be fully sustained by mitochondrial respiration is supplemented by anaerobic glycolysis and, in situations of a brief burst (as in a sprint), also by the stored phosphagen pool. The relative engagement of the anaerobic systems depends on the redox state of the cell, defined in simple terms by the NADH/NAD ratio or the ADP/ATP ratio. As both glycolysis and mitochondrial respiration are activated by ADP (the by-product of cross-bridge cycling), the rate of lactate formation is defined by power output and the magnitude of the energy demand above the peak rate at which mitochondria can oxidize the reducing equivalents (e.g. NADH) generated by glycolysis. Performance then is determined by the total ATP produced by both aerobic and anaerobic metabolic pathways. In events such as the 500 and 1000 m events, paddlers reach blood lactate levels of 12–14 mM, while in the canoe sprint slalom event, values of 16 mM have been recorded. The aim of training for the canoeist in events such as 500–1000 m events is to achieve the highest aerobic power possible above which glycolysis supplements ATP supply. While lactate accumulation is an indicator of anaerobic energy contribution, it does equate to lactate production, since considerably large amounts of lactate are taken up and oxidized to ATP by other muscles that are contracting submaximally (e.g. legs in canoeing), and by other organs such as the liver, brain, and heart. Lactate does not in itself cause fatigue but is a correlate of hydrogen ion production and inorganic phosphate accumulation, which are involved in muscle fatigue.

Efficiency

Excluding environmental conditions, gross mechanical efficiency is determined by the technical skill of the canoeist and drag, which is mainly defined by body mass and equipment technology. In kayaking, early reports on mechanical work recorded that the ratio of external stroke work performed that transmitted into boat propulsion was approximately 90% during a two-minute all-out performance simulating a 500 m race. *Mechanical efficiency* is defined as the ratio between mechanical work (mean power×time) and total energy expenditure (total heat produced+work performed). In general, the efficiency of oxidative phosphorylation is approximately 60% and excitation–contraction coupling is approximately 40%, resulting in an upper limit of efficiencies of approximately 24%. There is a paucity of data on efficiency in canoeing. Gross mechanical efficiency for other elite athletes (e.g. cyclists) is in the range of 18–24%. Mechanical efficiency can be routinely measured with accuracy during submaximal exercise using ergometers for indirect calorimetry, provided that the contribution of the anaerobic metabolism is negligible. Measures of efficiency during high-intensity exercise are technically difficult to determine due to the significant contribution of anaerobic pathways. This stems in part from the complexity of measuring energy expenditure (total enthalpy change) since the glycolytic and phosphagen contributions have different metabolic efficiencies. Simplified estimates of energy release by anaerobic energy pathways have been made by measuring the recovery VO_2 (oxygen debt) and blood lactate concentrations. Accurate measurements of aerobic and anaerobic energy expenditure are based on Fick-derived VO_2, lactate release across an exercising limb, and muscle biopsies for the measurement of change in muscle ATP, PCr, and lactate, along with accurate measures of muscle mass. The energy expenditure is then calculated as heat or the Gibbs free energy change per mole ATP utilized = 60 kJ; PCr hydrolyzed = 35 kJ; lactate formed = 65 kJ; and oxygen consumed = 52 kJ (at a P/O ratio of 2.5), although there is no full agreement on the exact free energy values of ATP hydrolysis that should be used in vivo. Another challenge is that muscle efficiency varies with the speed of muscle contraction and fiber type, with type I fibers being significantly more efficient. In other sports, it has been proposed that with long-term training, athletes may self-select duty cycles or cadences that approach individual maximal efficiencies. So far, the muscle efficiency measures and the trainability of efficiency remain to be explored in canoeing across racing distances from sprints to long distances. Optimization of cadence for high efficiencies for the individual athlete can be determined experimentally with the use of isokinetic ergometers, where the duty cycle can be kept constant while the resistance changes so that at every muscle length during the contraction, the load is exactly equal to the maximum tension the muscle can exert at that length.

Areas for future research

This brief review has focused on a summary of the primary physiological systems and bioenergetics of elite canoeing performance, including concepts covered in over 100 published papers on the topic. While a growing body of knowledge of physiological factors is emerging, more research on the physiology of performance in canoeing is needed. We conclude with a perspective on some suggested future directions for research that will add to a more comprehensive understanding of performance attributes that may guide scientific monitoring and training approaches in canoeing.

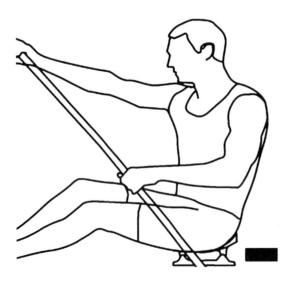

- Measures of mechanical efficiency (mechanical work per total energy expenditure) and contractile efficiency across distances of canoeing events
- Hemodynamics (blood flow), O_2 transport, and utilization in arms and legs during the canoe stroke
- The effect of entrainment on ventilatory mechanical restraint and the effect of inspiratory muscle training on performance
- The effect of dietary nutrients on metabolic function (e.g. bioenergetic efficiency of dietary beetroot, β-hydroxybutyrate)
- Identification of molecular biomarkers linked to the adaptive response to training (e.g., metabolomics, proteomics); optimization of the training dose
- Circadian rhythm, biological clock, training, and recovery and rest regimen.

Bibliography

Bishop, D. (2000). Physiological predictors of flat-water kayak performance in women. *Eur J Appl Physiol* 82 (1–2): 91–97.

Bonetti, D.L. and Hopkins, W.G. (2010). Variation in performance times of elite flat-water canoeists from race to race. *Int J Sports Physiol Perform* (2): 210–217.

Borges, G.F., Rama, L.M., Pedreiro, S. et al. (2012). Haematological changes in elite kayakers during a training season. *Appl. Physiol Nutrition Metab* 37 (6): 1140–1146.

Buglione, A., Lazzer, S., Colli, R. et al. (2011). Energetics of best performances in elite kayakers and canoeists. *Med Sci Sports Exerc* 43 (5): 877–884.

Byrnes, W.C. and Kearny, J.T. (1997). Aerobic and anaerobic contributions during simulated canoe/kayak events [Abstract]. *Med Sci Sports Exerc* 29: S220.

Clingeleffer, A., Mc Naughton, L., and Davoren, B. (1994). Critical power may be determined from two tests in elite kayakers. *Eur J Appl Physiol Occup Physiol* 68 (1): 36–40.

Fernandez, B., Perez-Landuce, J., Rodriguez, M., and Terrados, N. (1995). Metabolic contribution in Olympic kayaking events [Abstract]. *Med Sci Sports Exerc* 27: S24.

Forbes, S.C. and Chilibeck, P.D. (2007). Comparison of a kayaking ergometer protocol with an arm crank protocol for evaluating peak oxygen consumption. *J Strength Conditioning Res* 21 (4): 1282–1285.

Fry, R.W. and Morton, A.R. (1991). Physiological and kinanthropometric attributes of elite flatwater kayakists. *Med Sci Sports Exerc* 23 (11): 1297–1301.

García-Pallarés, J., García-Fernández, M., Sánchez-Medina, L., and Izquierdo, M. (2010a). Performance changes in world-class kayakers following two different training periodization models. *Eur J Appl Physiol* 110 (1): 99–107.

García-Pallarés, J. and Izquierdo, M. (2011). Strategies to optimize concurrent training of strength and aerobic fitness for rowing and canoeing. *Sports Med* 41 (4): 329–343.

Garcia-Pallares, J., Sanchez-Medina, L., Carrasco, L. et al. (2009). Endurance and neuromuscular changes in world-class level kayakers during a periodized training cycle. *Eur J Appl Physiol* 106 (4): 629–638.

Garcia-Pallares, J., Sanchez-Medina, L., Perez, C.E. et al. (2010b). Physiological effects of tapering and detraining in world-class kayakers. *Med Sci Sports Exerc* 42 (6): 1209–1214.

Gollnick, P.D., Armstrong, R.B., Saubert, C.W. et al. (1972). Enzyme activity and fiber composition in skeletal muscle of untrained and trained men. *J Appl Physiol* 33 (3): 312–319.

Gomes, B.B., Mourao, L., Massart, A. et al. (2012). Gross efficiency and energy expenditure in kayak ergometer exercise. *Intl J Sports Med* 33 (8): 654–660.

Kearny, J.T., and McKenzie, D. (2000) Physiology of canoe sport. In: Garrett, W., and Kirkendall, D.T. (eds.), *Exercise and sport science*. Philadelphia: Lippincott Williams & Wilkins.

Lundgren, K.M., Karlsen, T., Sandbakk, O. et al. (2015). Sport-specific physiological adaptations in highly trained endurance athletes. *Med Sci Sports Exerc* 47 (10): 2150–2157.

McKean, M.R. and Burkett, B.J. (2014). The influence of upper-body strength on flat-water sprint kayak performance in elite athletes. *Int J Sports Physiol Perform* 4: 707–714.

Michael, J.S., Rooney, K.B., and Smith, R. (2008). The metabolic demands of kayaking: a review. *J Sports Sci Med* 7 (1): 1–7.

Michael, J.S., Smith, R., and Rooney, K. (2010). Physiological responses to kayaking with a swivel seat. *Intl J Sports Med* 31 (8): 555–560.

Misigoj-Durakovic, M. and Heimer, S. (1992). Characteristics of the morphological and functional status of kayakers and canoeists. *J Sports Med Phys Fitness* 32 (1): 45–50.

Saltin, B. (1967). *Mexico City olympisk stad ett höjdfysiologiskt experiment*. Stockholm: Framtiden.

Saltin, B. and Astrand, P.O. (1967). Maximal oxygen uptake in athletes. *J Appl Physiol* 23 (3): 353–358.

Shephard, R.J. (1987). Science and medicine of canoeing and kayaking. *Sports Med* 4 (1): 19–33.

Tesch, P.A. (1983). Physiological characteristics of elite kayak paddlers. *Can J Appl Sport Sci* 8 (2): 87–91.

Tesch, P., Piehl, K., Wilson, G., and Karlsson, J. (1976). Physiological investigations of Swedish elite canoe competitors. *Med Sci Sports* 8 (4): 214–218.

Thomson, J.M. and Scrutton, E.W. (1978). Physiological adaptation to long-term upper-body work. *Can J Appl Sport Sci* 3 (2): 103–108.

van Someren, K.A. and Howatson, G. (2008). Prediction of flatwater kayaking performance. *Intl J Sports Physiol Perform* 3 (2): 207–218.

van Someren, K.A. and Palmer, G.S. (2003). Prediction of 200-m sprint kayaking performance. *Can J Appl Physiol* 28 (4): 505–517.

van Someren, K.A., Phillips, G.R., and Palmer, G.S. (2000). Comparison of physiological responses to open water kayaking and kayak ergometry. *Intl J Sports Med* 21 (3): 200–204.

Zamparo, P., Capelli, C., and Guerrini, G. (1999). Energetics of kayaking at submaximal and maximal speeds. *Eur J Appl Physiol Occup Physiol* 80 (6): 542–548.

Zamparo, P., Tomadini, S., Didonè, F. et al. (2006). Bioenergetics of a slalom kayak (k1) competition. *Int J Sports Med* 27 (7): 546–552.

Zouhal, H., Le Douairon Lahaye, S., Ben Abderrahaman, A. et al. (2012). Energy system contribution to Olympic distances in flat water kayaking (500 and 1,000 m) in highly trained subjects. *J Strength Condition Res* 26 (3): 825–831.

Chapter 5
Sport psychology for canoe and kayak

Penny Werthner

Faculty of Kinesiology, University of Calgary, Calgary, AB, Canada

Introduction

Winning an Olympic medal is the pinnacle of an athlete's career. However, it is an incredibly difficult task – to get everything right in a specific year, on a particular day, and at a precise time of day, in front of millions of people is an immense challenge. The pressure is considerable. So how does an athlete, and his or her coach, actually ensure that an optimal performance is achievable in such an environment? The answer is indeed quite complex, in part because there are a myriad of elements to consider and effectively manage, and, in part, because we are talking about human beings who themselves are quite complex.

The purpose of this chapter is to discuss the crucial psychological skills that must be developed to achieve an optimal performance at World Championships and Olympic Games. First, however, it is important to reflect briefly on the context of competitive sport and then explore the psychological elements in detail.

The elements of high-performance sport

One way to think about the context of competitive sport is as a number of critical elements that must all be taken care of to ensure success at the highest levels of sport. Coaches and athletes together must understand that these elements are closely interwoven.

The most significant element within the world of high-performance sport is certainly on the physiological side, which consists of training plans, technical training, strategy preparation, and so on. The second most important element could be termed *health considerations*, and this would include nutrition and injury prevention. The third element, specific to the sport of canoe and kayak, is equipment, more specifically the design of boats and paddles. A smaller, but not insignificant, element encompasses aspects such as socioculture, family, school, friends, and partners; and this element is psychological. It can be argued that while the physiological element is the most important during training phases, as the competition phase begins the

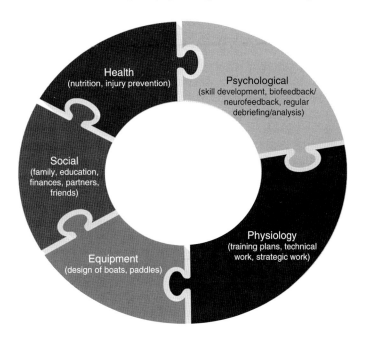

Figure 5.1 The elements of high-performance sport.

psychological aspect becomes more important. This is simply because competition is inherently stressful, and athletes need to develop the ability to manage such a stressful environment from a psychological perspective to perform optimally. Therefore, while taking into consideration all of these critical elements, athletes must prepare both physically and psychologically (Figure 5.1).

Psychological resilience and sport-specific psychological skills

There is a concept called *psychological resilience* that can be defined as the ability to adapt positively in the face of stress and adversity. Psychological resilience implies that an athlete has a level of self-confidence and optimism that helps them persevere in the face of the stress of high-performance competition. There is, of course, an ongoing discussion in the research literature about whether this concept of resilience is a trait (inherently who you are, your characteristics) or a state (a learned skill). There are certainly individual athletes who are inherently better able to cope with stress and adversity than others, but there is also considerable research support for the notion that most ath-

letes can learn to become stronger psychologically and therefore more psychologically resilient, and they do so through training specific psychological skills.

Within a strong body of research that has explored the importance of managing stress at the World Championship and Olympic level are a number of specific psychological skills that must be trained to provide an athlete with the opportunity to succeed and become consistently excellent in performance. And, importantly, just as physical training occurs on a daily basis throughout a training year, these skills must be practiced in a similar way.

The eight key psychological skills are the following abilities: *to develop a deep level of self-awareness, to focus on/concentrate on/"pay attention to" the correct cues at the correct time, to effectively manage arousal levels, to regularly debrief and analyze training and competition results, to effectively manage negative distractions, to set effective long- and short-term goals, to image and visualize,* and *to build an effective team culture in crew boats.* Each of these skills will be discussed in detail in this chapter. Also, the concept of *psychophysiology* will be introduced as an innovative method that enables athletes to learn how to effectively self-regulate.

Developing self-awareness: the learning process

A well-respected sport psychologist stated many years ago that sport psychology's motto is "Know thyself." Athletes and coaches must develop together an ability to become more deeply self-aware – developing a good sense of self-awareness and being honest with oneself are crucial underlying skills for competitive sport. Knowing what one is good at technically, tactically, strategically, and psychologically, and knowing what one needs to work on, are developed through regular dialogue during training sessions and regular analysis and a debriefing process after training sessions and critical competitions. This process, when done well, builds self-awareness and self-responsibility, creates a level of self-confidence, and ultimately ensures consistently good performances (Figure 5.2).

Developing the ability to focus and concentrate effectively

The skill of focus, or knowing what to concentrate on or "pay attention to," is a key psychological skill. Moran (2004) states that "concentration refers to a person's ability to exert deliberate mental effort on what is most important in any given situation" (p. 103), and it has been further described by direction (internal or external) and dimension (broad or narrow).

In sprint canoe and kayak, an effective focus is primarily achieved by creating a specific plan for each race, and in terms of direction and dimension it is internal and narrow. For example, in single kayak (K1) 200m, a plan would consist of a series of technical cues for the athlete to think about to stay focused on their own lane, in their own boat. This is an event of short duration, approximately 34 seconds, and there would not be too many cues. For example, a K1 200m plan might look like the following:

> Relaxed, top hand high, shoulders level
> Explosive, ready to go as gate drops
> Reach top speed at 50m
> Strong catch, each stroke
> Shoulders low, sit down
> Last 50m – keep up rate and rhythm
>> *(May also include a few confidence-building thoughts: "I have trained well," "I am ready," and "Just me, in my lane.")*

The primary purpose of such a plan is to ensure each athlete knows what to pay attention to or concentrate on that will enable his or her best race. Having a few specific cues to pay attention to

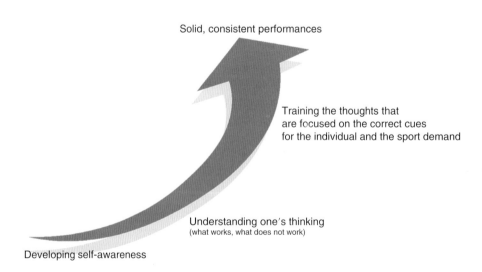

Figure 5.2 The process of learning in psychological skill development.

ensures that an athlete's mind has little time to dwell on any fears or concerns and all the negative possibilities. As well, to develop a viable plan requires a clear process. First, an initial plan needs to be developed; second, the plan needs to be trained in practice situations; third, the plan needs to be executed in a race situation as best as possible; fourth, a discussion needs to take place to analyze what occurred (the debrief); and then, fifth, the plan can be revised depending on the feedback from the coach, athlete, sport psychologist, and performance analyst. Importantly, this process creates an environment where an athlete regularly reflects on what works and what does not work for her or him – it is about discovering the right amount of cues. Too many cues are potentially overwhelming and can cause overthinking, but with too few, the potential for getting distracted by other competitors or a variety of other distractors is likely.

The skill of focus can also be practiced within training sessions by creating a clear purpose, or goal, for each week of practice and a daily goal for each day of practice – such as working on specific technique, times/splits, or the last 50 m/first 100 m of the race. Often, when athletes become skilled at their sport, they do not "need" to pay full attention to execute the skills in the training environment. This is understandable, and acceptable to a point, and it is undoubtedly important to not be overthinking. However, if an athlete does not practice, every day, being effectively focused in training, what often happens in competition is that he or she tries too hard and often overthinks on race day. It is a delicate balance, certainly – many athletes who are driven to excel overanalyze and think too much – so it is necessary that coach and athlete work on this together to find the right combination of cues, level of concentration, and just "letting it happen."

From a broader perspective, an athlete also requires a plan for the day of competition and, for example during Olympic Games, a plan for the 3 weeks in the Olympic village. Such *competition plans* ensure an athlete is organized, sleep is managed well, nutrition is taken care of, boat weighing is factored into the program, healthy distractions are planned (movies, time with family), training and taper are well planned, and recovery, both physiologically and psychologically, is taken into consideration.

A *race day plan* might look like the following:

Night before: Pack clothes (racing shirt, sunglasses, paddle, podium gear)
6:35 Alarm, out of bed, eat breakfast
8:00 Leave for course
8:30 On water warmup 1
8:50 Off water, rest
9:35 On water warmup 2
10:05 Race Final A, Lane X

Effectively managing arousal levels: finding the right intensity

A third key psychological skill for athletic performance is arousal control, and it has been noted that research on psychophysiological arousal and sport performance involves "highly variable terminology, such as arousal, alertness, vigilance and attention" (Bertollo et al. 2012, p. 92). In psychophysiological terms, *arousal* refers to the level of physiological activity and the "intensity" of behavior (Andreassi 2007). What is important in high-performance sport is to accept that competitive sport is inherently stressful. An athlete must first understand how he or she reacts to that stress, and what aspects are deemed negative; and, second, how "activated" or aroused he or she needs to be, which depends on what the event and sport demand, and, to a degree, on *who* the athlete is – is he or she more calm or more intense in day-to-day life? For example, from the perspective of what an event demands, an athlete competing in the single canoe (C1) or K1 200 m needs to be ready to be very explosive at the start, and activated; there is little room for error. In contrast, in K1 or C1/double canoe (C2) 1000 m, the crew or athlete needs to be ready for the first 250 m, they can be calmer due to the length of the race, but they must be prepared for the pain of the 1000 m that often begins after the first 250 m. The slalom paddler is exposed to a constant demand for technical excellence with little room for error. So, the objective is to be self-aware, know oneself, and know what is needed in the particular event. Ultimately, managing arousal levels is crucial for ensuring optimal performance because overarousal affects performance physically through increased muscle tension, fatigue, and movement impairment, and psychologically with an impairment of attention and focus. A number of studies have demonstrated improvements in athletes' arousal control through a variety of methods, including biofeedback, relaxation strategies, and progressive muscle relaxation. Biofeedback and its benefits will be discussed in greater detail later in this chapter.

Debriefing: effective analysis of training and performance results

Debriefing, or analysis of training and performances, is intended to be a process of self-reflection, which is defined by the *Merriam-Webster* dictionary as careful thought about one's own behaviors and beliefs. The process of debriefing with thorough analysis from a variety of perspectives is very much an opportunity for learning for both athletes and coaches. When the process is conducted effectively, it creates an environment for objective discussion about progress and results, ensures an athlete learns and grows as both a high-performance athlete and an individual, results in greater accountability, and, most notably, greatly improves the possibility for better performances. Each training period or race debrief provides an opportunity to help an athlete increase self-awareness and take greater responsibility for his or her performance. At the end of any debriefing meeting, the athlete should be clear on their progression, how they are doing relative to seasonal performance goals, and action steps for the next phase of training and competing.

The process of regular debriefing or analysis also results in psychological recovery. It is important to analyze good performances as well as suboptimal performances, but it is the latter that, more often than not, elicits strong emotional responses – sadness, disappointment, anger, and despair – and it is important that the athlete is able to talk about those negative emotions, to ensure she or he does not get "stuck" in them. With an effective analysis or debriefing process, an athlete can express those emotions, reflect on what occurred, begin to learn from any mistakes, and begin to create a new plan

for the next competition. Similarly, if the performance or training block was very good, it is important to discuss how and why it was good, so the learning reaffirms good behaviors.

Creating a regular process of debriefing/analysis can involve both informal and formal processes. First, from a more informal perspective, it is possible to think about debriefing/analysis as simply a discussion between a coach and an athlete about how daily training is going, how fatigue levels are, what is happening in life outside sport, and what might need to be adjusted. The more formal process could consist of three kinds of meetings: (i) a meeting for debrief/assessment/analysis of each racing weekend; (ii) a midpoint debrief/assessment/analysis of the year to date – for canoe and kayak, that might be midpoint of the summer season; and (iii) a year-end review, which would involve the athlete's perspective, the coach's perspective, and the sport science team's perspective, if other individuals are working with the athlete or crew. Finally, it is important to consider the timing of when a debrief takes place. For example, if it is a race being debriefed and the performance is suboptimal, the athlete will likely be emotional, and it would be best to wait until after a warmdown is completed. It could also wait until the next day, but it is important that the discussion take place within a day or two of the event so that the details can be recalled vividly.

A word of caution – in the beginning, athletes may not always have the capacity to self-reflect effectively and objectively. Developing an effective analysis process requires gentleness, a gathering of facts from training or performance, and good questions such as "Let's talk about today's race: tell me what you thought?" and "Tell me how that second 250 was – what were you thinking and feeling at that point?" What is most important is creating an environment where the athlete feels safe enough to reflect honestly on what occurred in the race (Figure 5.3).

Effectively managing negative distractions

In high-performance sport, there are many distractions that can take an athlete away from their best focus or effective state of concentration. In the

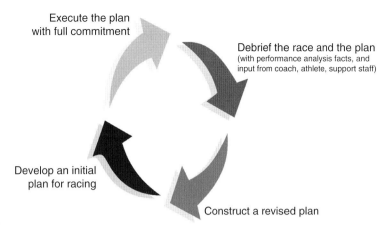

Figure 5.3 Debrief process.

sport of canoe and kayak, there may be external negative distractions such as poor water conditions, rain and wind, an inconsistent starter, a delay in start times, or an equipment problem. There can also be numerous internal distractions such as a fear of losing, anxiety around making a final, expectations created internally, and numerous unproductive thoughts such as "I need to be in the top three to qualify for the championships" "Can I do this?" "What if my training was not right?" or "I never do well in these conditions."

One of the best ways to prepare for these negative distractions is to create a list of all the possible negative distractions that might occur, and then a second list of the solutions to each of the distractions – understanding that many negative distractions can be controlled (e.g. one's own thoughts, or one's reaction to the starter) but others are not controllable (e.g. weather conditions or a delay in starting time). Nevertheless, it is important that athletes learn that they always have a *choice* in how they react to a situation. Learning to effectively focus and refocus on the correct cues, in the face of negative distractions, is always a choice.

Setting effective long- and short-term goals

A goal is an objective standard, or the aim of some action. Subjective goals are more general statements of intent, such as "I want to enjoy my sport" or "I want to do my best"; objective goals may be more general, such as making a team, or

more specific, such as working to become more skilled at paddling in crew boats.

There are three types of objective goals that an athlete can work with – outcome goals, performance goals, and process goals. An *outcome goal* emphasizes a focus on results, such as winning a race, and often depends on others. A *performance goal* emphasizes achieving a standard based on the athlete's previous performance. This is a more internal goal. A *process goal* emphasizes actions an athlete will engage in during a performance to execute or perform well, such as a solid top hand, power on each stroke, and focus on good catch. All three types of goals are important and should be written down, revisited regularly through the debriefing process, and adjusted as needed. It is important to create goals, or a purpose, for each week of training that are realistic and challenging at the same time. When realistic and measurable goals are set, they can be assessed accurately, and when a goal is achieved, it is incredibly motivating for an athlete. Therefore, setting lots of small, measurable, daily process goals and committing to them provide an athlete with the best chance for building self-confidence and improvement in competition.

It is also essential to understand that while all three kinds of goals are important, outcome goals often become a very real stressor for most athletes close to a competition because the outcome (winning a race, beating competitors, or winning a World Championship or an Olympic medal) is not within one's direct control. Close to competition and on competition day, process goals are the best because they are closely linked to an effective focus, directing an athlete's attention to what they can control – how he or she will move the boat – regardless of what their competitors might be doing.

Visualization: our mind's eye

Visualization is the seventh psychological skill that is necessary to develop. The images can be visual ("seeing" how a race might unfold, or how a specific technique can be executed), auditory ("hearing" the sounds of the paddle in the water or teammates along the course), kinesthetic ("feeling" the movement in the boat), and/or olfactory (the "smell" of the competition site). There are also two types of imagery – internal (where an athlete images the execution of a skill from his or her own vantage point) and external (where an athlete sees himself or herself executing the skill, as in watching a video). There is an ongoing discussion in the research literature, but no definitive conclusions, on which perspective is more effective. What is most important is that athletes develop an ability to "see" and "feel" correct execution of skills, their role on the crew boat, and their plan for racing, and develop the ability to be consciously in control of the imagery.

When imagery or visualization is practiced regularly, it can build confidence, enhance motivation, speed up motor learning, and complement the physical practice of specific skills. To become better at this skill, the first step for an athlete is to "remember" or re-create in her or his mind a positive past performance or technical aspect that he or she already does well. When beginning to learn this skill, it is easier to visualize something that one already does well. A second step occurs when the athlete has developed an ability to image past events: he or she can begin to "image" or see/feel a future event, such as next month's World Championships – what the venue looks like, how they want to race, and what they want to focus on – and visualize the plan for racing. Most importantly, the visualization should always be positive – for example, the athlete sees and feels herself or himself successfully executing the skill or the race.

Building an effective team culture in crew boats

A *team* has been defined as any group of people who must interact with each other to accomplish shared objectives. Great performances happen in crew boats when an athlete feels a sense of team. When athletes are able to move from a group of individuals with a focus on themselves to a crew where there is a common goal and an emphasis on executing each respective role in the boat, the chances of success increase. To build such a crew boat requires time in the boat, a clear set of long- and short-term daily goals, clarity on one's "job" in the boat, clarity and commitment to the plan for racing, and debriefs after each training session and each race, where each of the athletes reflects on how it went and provides suggestions for improvement on training aspects and on the plan for the next race. In this process, it is important that the athletes speak first, and then the coach can add his or her perspective, with any video analysis and notes acting as the factual information. This builds accountability and personal responsibility. It is important again to discuss both what went poorly and what went well, and end the discussion with a few action steps for each athlete. This kind of discussion with crew boat members requires excellent communication skills to manage the inevitable conflicts that will arise. In many cases, it will take a season or two to get a crew working well together and solidify a plan for racing that is understood and accepted for each member of the crew, and numerous races at top speed to be assured that the crew can race successfully and consistently at an optimal level.

Psychophysiology: the use of bio- and neurofeedback

In discussing the key psychological skills, it is understood that these skills, when well learned, help an athlete manage the demands of the stressful environment of high-performance sport. Psychophysiological training – specifically, the use of bio- and neurofeedback – is a methodology designed to help athletes learn to self-regulate on multiple levels (i.e. psychologically, emotionally, and physiologically).

Bio- and neurofeedback training, or psychophysiological training, involves the development of a deep self-awareness and self-regulation of both physiological and neurological activity in the body and brain. It is designed to enhance an athlete's awareness of, and ability to influence and control, her or his optimal performance state. Bio- and neurofeedback is based on the underlying principle that the nervous system is the command center of the body. The nervous system is divided into two parts: the central nervous system and the peripheral nervous system. Information travels within and among the two divisions via neural tissue. The central nervous system includes the brain and spinal cord. The peripheral nervous system has two divisions: somatic (voluntary) and autonomic (involuntary).

Biofeedback training targets the autonomic nervous system, which consists of the sympathetic nervous system, which activates the fight-or-flight response in the body (the stress response); and the parasympathetic nervous system, which deactivates the fight-or-flight response in the body and allows the body to rest and regenerate (the relaxation response). When an athlete experiences anxiety or stress, the sympathetic nervous system becomes dominant. The purpose of the biofeedback training is to enable each athlete to improve the balance between sympathetic and parasympathetic nervous system activity.

Biofeedback training includes several forms of feedback, including electromyography (EMG), electrodermal activity (EDA), peripheral body temperature, heart rate (HR), and respiration rate and depth. Specifically, the feedback provides an athlete with visual information about his or her physiological responses, and therefore enables the athlete to learn to self-regulate arousal levels.

Neurofeedback, or electroencephalography (EEG) biofeedback, provides information on the athlete's cortical activity, which is measured in various frequencies ranging from delta (associated with deep sleep) to theta (daydreaming), alpha (readiness state), low beta (focused attention), and high beta (worry and rumination). During training, athletes receive visual and/or auditory feedback and are encouraged to enhance low beta for focused attention and limit both theta (daydreaming) and high beta (rumination and anxiety). This training provides the athlete with self-regulation skills enabling him or her to effectively focus on the task at hand.

There is a body of research on both biofeedback and neurofeedback and sport, but to date, from a neurofeedback perspective, only closed-skill, self-paced sport athletes (marksmanship, archery, and golf) have been measured during actual physical performance. To date, EEG equipment has been such that minimal movement affects the EEG signal. However, new equipment is being developed and trialed that may allow for accurate measurement of EEG with movement.

In summary, the development and continual fine-tuning of these eight psychological skills – and, if possible, the use of psychophysiological training (using bio- and neurofeedback) – enable an athlete to develop a deep sense of self-awareness, a solid level of self-confidence, and the psychological resilience necessary to cope effectively with the stress and demands of training and competition within the world of high-performance sport. It is important to remember that these skills must be practiced regularly, in both training sessions and in competition; and, to learn effectively and progress, a regular process of self-reflection and debriefing must occur.

Bibliography

Andreassi, J.L. (2007). *Psychophysiology: human behavior and physiological response*, 5th edn. Mahwah, NJ: Lawrence Erlbaum.

Bertollo, M., Robazza, C., Falasca, W.N. et al. (2012). Temporal pattern of pre-shooting psychophysiological states in elite athletes: a probabilistic approach. *Psych Sport Exerc* 13: 91–98.

Blumenstein, B., Bar-Eli, M., and Tenenbaum, G. (2002). *Brain and body in sport and exercise: biofeedback applications in performance enhancement*. New York: Wiley.

Davis, P., Sime, W.E., and Robertson, J. (2007). Sport psychophysiology and peak performance applications of stress management. In: *Principles and practice of stress management*, 3rd edn (ed. P.M. Lehrer, W.E. Sime and R.L. Woolfolk), 615–637. New York: Guilford Press.

Dupee, M. and Werthner, P. (2011). Managing the stress response: the use of biofeedback and neurofeedback with Olympic athletes. *Biofeedback* 39: 92–94.

Dupee, M., Werthner, P., and Forneris, T. (2015). A preliminary study on the relationship between athletes' ability to self-regulate and world ranking. *Biofeedback* 43 (2): 57–63.

Galloway, S.M. (2011). The effect of biofeedback on tennis service accuracy. *Intl J Sport Exerc Psych* 9: 251–266.

Gould, D., Dieffenbach, K., and Moffett, A. (2002). Psychological characteristics and their development in Olympic champions. *J Appl Sport Psych* 14 (3): 172–204.

Jones, G., Hanton, S., and Connaughton, D. (2007). A framework of mental toughness in the world's best performers. *Sport Psychologist* 21 (2): 243–264.

Moran, A. (2004). *Sport and exercise psychology: a critical introduction*. London: Routledge.

Oudejans, R., Kuijpers, W., Kooijman, C., and Bakker, F. (2011). Thoughts and attention of athletes under pressure: skill-focus or performance worries? *Anxiety Stress Coping* 24 (1): 59–73.

Reeves, C., Nicholls, A., and McKenna, T. (2011). The effects of a coping intervention on coping self-efficacy, coping effectiveness, and subjective performance among adolescent soccer players. *Intl J Sport Exerc Psych* 9 (2): 126–142.

Robazza, C., Pellizzari, M., Bertollo, M., and Hanin, Y.L. (2008). Functional impact of emotions on athletic performance: comparing the IZOF model and the directional perception approach. *J Sports Sci* 26 (10): 1033–1047.

Werthner, P., Christie, S., and Dupee, M. (2013). Neurofeedback and biofeedback training with Olympic athletes. *NeuroConnections* 2: 32–37.

Chapter 6
Training for canoeing

Martin Hunter[1] and Sylvain Curinier[2–4]

[1]Swedish Canoe Federation, Rosvalla, Sweden

[2]Fédération Française de Canoë-Kayak (FFCK), Joinville-le-Pont, France

[3]INSEP, Paris, France

[4]France PNL, Paris, France

SECTION 1: SPRINT

Martin Hunter
Swedish Canoe Federation, Rosvalla, Sweden

Introduction

The competition season, and specifically the more important events for an athlete, should be the starting point for the planning of the training of an athlete. For elite athletes, this will be either the World Championships or Olympic Games, depending on the year. This is the case for both sprint canoeing and slalom canoeing, as both are included in the Olympic Games program.

Planning involves working backward from the penultimate goal and periodizing the athlete's plan. Part of this plan should include the different physiological aspects, such as aerobic and anaerobic capacity, strength training, sports science, and psychology. The long-term (two to five years) and short-term (less than two years) goals will also be partially determined by the athlete's economic and social situation (do they have work, family, etc.). Geographical aspects will also impact the planning; for example, can an athlete train all year-round, or are the lakes frozen for half of the year?

Now that the 200 m event has been included in the Olympic program, there are three distinct groups of athletes. The first is the 1000 m group (TMG), which has a more traditional planning structure; the second group is the 200 m group, which has a greater focus on anaerobic and power development; and the third group, the women's group, has a mixture of aerobic and anaerobic capacities. The women race 200 and 500 m events, so the contrast between groups is not as significant as in the men's group. However, we are seeing more and more that women specialize in a particular event.

Many countries have produced documentation in the form of requirements plans, describing what an athlete needs to do if they wish to become competitive at an elite level. These documents can also be used as a guideline when planning training.

Section 1 of the chapter will outline the planning process, then will suggest the type, amount, and when each particular aspect of the program should be implemented, and why. It will focus on senior sprint athletes, not junior athletes.

The planning process

The planning process should start by looking at the individual athlete and what they need. Begin the process by looking at the strengths and weaknesses,

Canoeing, First Edition. Edited by Don McKenzie and Bo Berglund.
© 2019 International Olympic Committee. Published 2019 by John Wiley & Sons Ltd.

and opportunities and threats, associated with a particular athlete.

Strengths: What is the athlete good at? Do they have the financial support; what about support from friends and family? Maybe the athlete is very good at particular activities – is he or she very explosive? Many factors need to be considered at this stage.

Weaknesses: Is the athlete capable of managing the training program? Does the athlete have shoulder problems? Is he or she psychologically weak? If an athlete is overly focused, this could be seen as a weakness.

Opportunities: An athlete may receive sponsorship, which will enable them to pursue their sport fully, and not have to worry about financial aspects. Training with athletes that are better or much better than them is an important opportunity. In this case, the coach must coordinate the training with these athletes. The short-term benefits of training with a faster athlete will most probably outweigh training alone!

Threats: These could include possible injuries or financial problems. For example, does the athlete have the financial resources to do the training, buy the necessary equipment, and train the necessary

quantity in the time available? Do they work full time, for example?

Many of the factors involved in the planning process are summarized in Figure 6.1. There are many different factors that go into this process, and Figure 6.1 shows that one of the most important aspects to be considered and understood is what the athlete wants. Often, conflict may occur if the coach's expectations and demands do not match up with the needs and wants of the athlete.

What type of training?

To be the best in canoeing or kayaking, the athlete should train as much as possible in that particular boat as opposed to using a paddling ergometer. Training will also be affected by many variables, such as time (does the athlete have the time with study and work to complete full sessions?) and geography (e.g. where temperatures or conditions make it impossible to train). Many different models of paddling ergometers are available, and the athlete will most likely have their own particular preference.

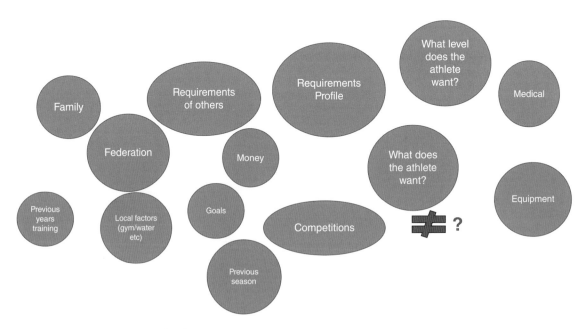

Figure 6.1 Factors involved in the planning process.

Other forms of training that are recommended are bike riding (which has similar motions to kayaking, with both push and pull with legs and arms), running (the simplest alternative), and cross-country skiing (which is regarded as being excellent for improving maximal aerobic capacity). Swimming is often considered an excellent form of cross-training. The benefit of swimming is that it is regarded as a low-impact sport, as the water is regarded as a "soft" medium.

Strength is enhanced by training in the gym, using weights. Predominantly, free weights are used, but machines are also used. Strength training will be discussed in more detail further into this chapter.

Aerobic and anaerobic capacity

Kayak speed is determined by a number of factors, and it can be subdivided into two major groups – the equipment and the physiology of the athlete. Kayaks have developed considerably from the early Olympic examples, which were made of wood and canvas. Today's kayaks are made of carbon fiber, and some are even "tuned" to suit individual kayakers' technique and body mass, using accelerometer and GPS technology. All kayaks race at a standard weight, depending on class. Paddles have developed from soft, flat wooden paddles to hard, wing-shaped carbon fiber paddles, which have been reported to increase efficiency by 74–89% when compared to the traditional "flat" paddle. The forces acting on the kayak are both aerodynamic (above the waterline) and hydrodynamic (below the waterline – including friction/surface tension, pressure or form drag, and wave drag), and these must be overcome to move the kayak through the water.

The physiological factors needed to maximize the velocity of the kayak include the ability to generate high average power, the ability to create large average forces, effective technical skills, and a large metabolic capacity. It has been suggested that a change of 0.3–0.6% in performance time, or a 1–2% increase in power output from one season to the next, is needed to improve medal prospects in flat-water kayak racing. In elite sport, margins of winning are becoming

smaller and smaller. Elite athletes and their coaches are looking for ways to improve performance.

Some of the more common tests used to monitor an athlete's performance levels include tests for aerobic power ($\dot{V}o_2max$): the highest rate of oxygen consumption attainable during maximal or exhaustive exercise; and aerobic capacity: the ability to work at a given workload for a longer time. Aerobic power can be described as the body's ability to create energy per time interval through the use of oxygen. Healthy humans, irrespective of sex, age, or fitness level, will have maximal oxygen consumption of between 2 and 6L of oxygen per minute. Aerobic capacity is the ability to develop energy from aerobic processes for a longer work time. With a high aerobic capacity, an individual can have higher relative work intensity when compared to another individual with a lower capacity, that is, the ability to work at a higher percentage of $\dot{V}O_2max$.

By tradition, aerobic power or $\dot{V}o_2max$ has been considered as one of the most important measures for assessing the potential for endurance performance. $\dot{V}O_2max$ has been defined as the highest rate of oxygen consumption attainable during maximal or exhaustive exercise. It occurs when there is a plateau in the oxygen consumption curve even as work rate continues to increase. $\dot{V}O_2max$ is defined as the highest value of oxygen consumption measured during a graded exercise test. The factors that can affect the amount of maximal oxygen uptake are both central and peripheral in nature. The *central factors* include (i) the pulmonary diffusing capacity, (ii) maximal cardiac output, and (iii) the oxygen carrying capacity of the blood. The *peripheral factors* refer to the skeletal muscle characteristics and would include increased muscle capillarization, increased intramuscular mitochondrial density, and increased percentage of type 1 fibers. Studies have shown that Olympic kayak paddlers need a high aerobic capacity, as well as a high aerobic power contribution. For the purpose of this chapter, $\dot{V}o_2max$ refers to kayak or kayak ergometer $\dot{V}o_2max$ values. The Swedish Canoe Federation's official documentation, Kravanalys ("requirements profile"), suggests that elite athletes, if they are to be considered medal prospects, are required to have values for $\dot{V}o_2peak$ of 4.9, 5.4, and 5.6 L·min^{-1} for 200, 500, and 1000 m, respectively.

Many different names and terminology are used to define aerobic capacity. For example, commonly used terminology includes the anaerobic threshold, the onset of blood lactate accumulation (OBLA), maximal lactate steady state (MLSS), and individual lactate threshold. Anaerobic threshold is a concept, and definitions are conceptual definitions. During steady-state exercise, the aerobic metabolism matches the energy requirements of the active muscles. It is the level at which oxygen uptake cannot account for all the required energy needed for that exercise intensity. Lactate production matches the lactate consumption, or, put another way, the rate of appearance equals the rate of disappearance. The lactate threshold is the highest oxygen consumption or exercise intensity achieved with less than a $1.0\,mmol·L^{-1}$ increase in blood lactate concentration above the pre-exercise level. Onset of blood lactate accumulation (OBLA) occurs when the blood lactate concentration increases to $4.0\,mmol·L^{-1}$. This is the maximal intensity that can be maintained for a prolonged time. There is agreement that the $4.0\,mmol·L^{-1}$ level of blood lactate is associated with the lactate threshold and is an important factor in endurance performance. In a study of a group ($n = 16$) of well-trained 3000 m runners, it was found that the running velocity at OBLA explained the large variability in the running performance.

Training intensities

Training intensities described in this chapter are based on the Swedish standard, and they are similar in different countries but with minor variations. Depending on the influence of the sport scientist and on how the coach writes the training program, intensities can be described in different ways. For example, it may be easier to write a program that is based on speed (athletes use GPS/SpeedCoach®), as suggested in Table 6.1.

Note that in Table 6.1, the lactate levels are only a guide; variations occur in different individuals and can change over time. For athlete A, this might mean a heart rate of 140±5 beats; for athlete B, it could be 145±5 beats. The coach should ask for this to be specified by the sport scientist. Generally, however, the speed on the water is similar for all

Table 6.1 Speed comparisons for training purposes based on 500 m times.

Minute	Seconds	Total seconds	m s^{-1}	km h^{-1}	% of Maximum	Intensity
1	32.5	92.50	5.4	19.5	104	5
1	35.0	95.00	5.3	18.9	102	5
1	37.5	97.50	5.1	18.5	100	4
1	40.0	100.00	5.0	18.0	98	4
1	42.5	102.50	4.9	17.6	95	4
1	45.0	105.00	4.8	17.1	93	4
1	47.5	107.50	4.7	16.7	91	4
1	50.0	110.00	4.5	16.4	89	3
1	52.5	112.50	4.4	16.0	87	3
1	55.0	115.00	4.3	15.7	85	3
1	57.5	117.50	4.3	15.3	83	3
1	60.0	120.00	4.2	15.0	81	3

For example: An athlete's best time over 500 m is 1 minute 40 seconds. Thus, a lactate threshold training program for 10*500 m could be written as:
10*500 @85% *or*
10*500 @4.3 m/s *or*
10*500 @ intensity 3 *or*
10*500 @ 140±5 BPM
This is actually a good way to bring variety into the training program.
BPM, Heartbeats per minute.

Table 6.2 Training intensities.

Intensity	Heart rate (% of maximum)	Lactate (mmol L⁻¹)
5	90–100%	>10
4	90–100%	6–9
3+	90–95%	4–6 (3–8)
3	80–90%	4 (2–6)
2	60–75%	2–3
1	50–60%	<2

Source: Svenska Kanotförbundet (2009).

athletes at the different speeds at the elite level. Therefore, the individual should be tested regularly. The base guideline for the relationship between speed and lactate levels is suggested in Table 6.2.

Strength training

Which exercises, how often, how many reps, and how many sets are questions frequently discussed and argued about. To understand what should be trained in the gym, it is important to have an understanding of canoeing technique, as well as how the effect of the paddle causes the boat to move through the water.

Strength is of vital importance to performance of the athlete. The boat weighs 12 kg, there is resistance of the water, and it is the blade that is the final factor in transmitting all the power to the water.

Development of power in four-person kayak (K4) is of even more importance, as the boat weighs 32 kg, plus the weight of the other athletes. Thus, to move the boat past the paddle, great force must be created.

How strong should you be? Suggested strength demands as suggested by the Swedish KravAnalys are shown in Table 6.3.

Can an athlete be too strong? This was starting to become a problem before the introduction of carbon fiber paddles. With this change, the shafts on paddles are now almost unbreakable. Specificity of strength is important. The athlete may be able to lift huge weights, but if they are not able to translate this to the water, then it will be of no use. The possible by-product of becoming too strong would be that the athlete could lose flexibility or range of movement.

The next section will look at both technique and the movement of the paddle in the water.

Canoeing technique

To simplify the technique to a simple and understandable level, the technique used in kayak racing has been broken down into four phases:

1 *Entry into the water*: The paddle enters the water, then starts the movement to propel the canoe. Also called the *entry phase*.

Table 6.3 Strength demands: kayak.

Strength type/exercise	Men's 1000 m	Women's 500 and 200 m	Men's 200 m
Maximum Strength			
Bench Press (1RM)	>1.4 × Bodyweight	>1.1–1.2 × Bodyweight	>1.8 × Bodyweight
Bench Pull (1RM)	>1.2–1.3 × Bodyweight	>1.0 × Bodyweight	>1.8 × Bodyweight
Chins with weight (1RM)	>50 kg	>25 kg	>70 kg
Dips with weight (1RM)	>50 kg	>35 kg	>70 kg
Strength Endurance			
BP 2 minutes 55 kg M/40 kg W	>100	>80	>100
Bench Pulls 2 minutes 55 kg M/40 kg W	>100	>80	>100
Chins	>35	>35	>35
Dips	>35	>25	>35

Source: Svenska Kanotförbundet (2009). Modified by the author.

2 *Moving through the water*: This is a misnomer of the aim of this phase – the paddle in fact should be relatively stationary, and the boat should be moving past the paddle (especially as speeds become higher). Also called the *pull phase*.

3 *Exit from water*: Also called the *exit phase*.

4 *Movement though the air*: Also called the *air phase*.

Biomechanical performances of paddles

In each of these phases, different muscles are involved, but by having a basic understanding of technique, it is possible to identify the major groups and forces involved. Results from biomechanical tests show that the peak force is produced approximately one-third of the way through the stroke. It is reasonable to assume that this is a result of the actual blade taking time to become efficient in the water. Peak force on a paddle machine occurs much sooner, and it is most likely the result of the gearing and mechanical advantages of the machine itself, as there is a significant mechanical and hydrodynamic advantage as opposed to the blade in the water.

The factors that affect the biomechanical performance in paddling are as follows:

1 Peak power
2 Impulse
3 Stroke rate
4 The total time that the blades are in the water (TBW = time blade in water)
5 Percentage of the stroke cycle that the paddle is in the water
6 Speed of the kayak
7 Instantaneous changes in velocity.

Peak power

The importance of peak power becomes obvious when the paddle is in the water. Generally, the greater the peak power that the athlete can produce, the greater the potential to create a higher impulse, assuming that the time in which the power is produced is constant. Thus, with kayaking, it is important to find a good balance between one's strength and bodyweight. An increase in bodyweight will result in greater resistance of the boat in the water, which in turn will demand a more effective use of the musculature in relation to power development and speed. Increased weight as the result of increased muscle mass does not necessarily produce negative consequences; on the contrary, if this muscle can be used in an effective way, it is beneficial.

Impulse and frequency (stroke rate)

Impulse is calculated by multiplying the power produced by the time the power is in effect (the time it is in the water). Frequency in canoeing is the stroke rate per minute. The relationship between impulse and frequency is very important in sprint, as these two factors determine how much work is produced. Work, in turn, is that factor that is responsible for moving the boat through the water.

TBW and the percentage of time the paddle is in the water

A higher stroke rate will automatically result in a higher percentage of the time the blade is in the water. This can be a little difficult to understand, as a higher frequency will result in a reduced TBW, but in relation to the stroke cycle's air phase (when the paddle is in the air), TBW is reduced only marginally. Therefore, the percentage of the time the paddle is in the water during a full stroke cycle increases, even if the TBW is reduced when stroke rate is increased.

The optimal interval for the time that the paddle should be in the water is considered to be between 67 and 75%. Values that are under 67% are believed to influence speed variations and thus decrease the physical effect. Values over 75% will result in the time between strokes being so small that it will lead to faster exhaustion, loss of technique, and greater lactic acid production. Once one understands the effects of the paddle in the water and the canoeing technique, it is possible to determine the muscles used.

Designing the complete training program

Once the coach has a basic understanding of the technique and physiological aspects of the sport of canoeing, the coach can start to plan the training.

Yearly plan

The best plan to start with is a year's or season's plan (e.g. from World Championship to World Championship). In this plan, you would start by putting in all the competitions, then other important events affecting training, such as training camps and other meetings.

It is suggested that a stepped structure be followed for the weekly plan. Should the week be an easy week, medium week, or hard week? For example, weeks 1–5 could be easy, medium, medium hard, hard, and easy, respectively. In this way, it is possible to build progression into the training plan.

It is important to point out that a yearlong plan will be a living document, which will need to be updated and modified as the season continues. Changes to the plan could result from changes in the competition calendar, athlete injury, change in focus for a particular athlete, or any number of other factors.

Designing a weekly training program

Once a plan for the year is done, the weekly plan can be developed. From the year's plan, you will know the week's focus, amount of kilometers desired, number of gym sessions and type of gym, and other relevant information. The plan can be written as follows:

1 Write in where you want the rest or supercompensation session, usually Wednesday or Thursday afternoon. This way, there can be a similar number of sessions early in the week as there are after.

2 Plan the gym sessions. Three per week, spread over Monday, Wednesday, and Friday, are commonly accepted as being best. You could, however, have three per week and four the next (Monday, Wednesday, Friday, Sunday, Tuesday, Thursday, Saturday, and so on).

3 Plan the paddling sessions and the particular boat (K1, K2, K4, C1, or C2)

4 Once you have all these data, the different sessions can be designed. For example, now you will be able to add the aerobic and anaerobic sessions, as well as recovery sessions.

5 The actual choice of session will then be up to the coach, and will be based on the requirements of that particular training cycle. The focus is on improving speed, speed endurance, and aerobic or anaerobic capacity. The suggested rule is to calculate the effective time in each session, at a particular intensity. One should also look at recovery time between particular sessions. For example, a shorter speed session would need less recovery time afterward compared to a longer aerobic session. To put a speed session or even a technique session after a heavy gym session would not be advised, as the wrong muscle groups would be used, and in the case of a technique session, it would not be possible to maintain proper technique if you were tired.

6 The coach should then implement the program, and being willing and flexible during the week if any modifications to the program are to be conducted.

7 Monitoring the athlete's development will also be an important part of the plan. Thus, regular gym tests (suggested every 6 weeks) and on-water tests are recommended to be conducted. An example gym test is included later in the chapter.

Strength training

Based on knowledge of the musculature used in the canoeing stroke, it is possible to simplify the training regime into push-and-pull exercises. Thus, to design a gym program, the coach needs to understand what event the athlete will compete in, and then design the program around this based on the yearly plan for training. Normally, it is accepted to periodize the strength training into 4- to 6-week periods with a particular focus in mind, for example maximum strength.

The trend nowadays has been to get the athlete to train many Olympic lifts to teach the body how to work effectively as a whole. This may be the case, but there is no getting away from the need to be strong enough in the sport-specific exercises used in canoeing. There is also no scientific documentation or studies to show that this is beneficial to the sport of canoeing. Time is often limited, so an athlete must make the best of this time. For example, if a female canoeist cannot do more chin-ups than, say, 10 reps, then it would be more beneficial for her to focus on training chins instead of snatches or cleans.

Examples of the different foci in strength training are shown in Table 6.4. The table also shows the set and reps for each particular type of training.

Training program examples

Week 7 training: Florida, USA

Week 7		Session	Comments	Area to focus on	Specific focus
Monday	AM	Gym Program 1	Stretching after session		Speed, max strength, endurance strength, coordination, flexibility
	FL	10 km 2 km easy, 7 km@2, 1@1		Focus on placing the blade in the water	Technique, coordination
	PM	10*4@3–3+		AT	Technique, coordination
Tuesday	AM				
	FL	10*750@3	Technique with hard starts	Start phase to transition	Explosiveness, speed, technique, coordination
	PM	10*1000@ 200 splits speed 3/4	K2	Boat run and boat control	Technique, coordination/ timing
Wednesday	AM	Gym Program 2			
	FL	Easy 10 km			
	PM	10*30/30, 15*10/10	All efforts should be races; win as many as possible	Speed endurance and speed when the athlete is tired. Mental aspect is also worked.	Speed endurance, lactate tolerance, mental tolerance
Thursday	AM	Rest			
	PM	1*500, 1*1000	Time trials: usual race warmup.	Testing new race plans	A test of all factors
Friday	AM	Gym Program 3			Max strength, coordination
	FL	5 km resistance with 2*5 starts right/left	Directly after gym; sea anchor or tennis ball resistance		Specific strength
	PM	25 km (5*2, 5@3, 3@4, 2@2, 5@3)			Endurance
Saturday	AM	Mini Triathlon (Swim 3, Run 10 km. Paddle 15 km)	All start together.		Endurance, aerobic capacity
	PM	Off			
Sunday	AM	Rest Day all day	Try to find something to do to get the athletes away from home!	Some light stretching	Recovery

AM, Before breakfast; FL, before lunch; PM, afternoon.

Table 6.4 Sets, reps, and intensity.

MS	Maximum strength: 3–5 sets × 1–3 reps (rest 3–5 minutes) MS 85–100% or 1 RM
ES	Explosive strength: 3–6 sets with 4–6 reps (rest between 2 and 5 minutes) ES 70–85% of 1 RM
SS	Speed strength: 3–6 sets × 6–10 reps (high speed of movement, rest between 2 and 4 SS minutes)
MSS	Maximum speed: (60–85% of 1 RM) 1–3 sets × 5–6 reps (long rest, max speed of movement)
E	Endurance: 2–4 sets × 15–50 reps (rest 1–2 minutes) E
ANE	Anaerobic endurance: long time intervals/high reps, 1–5 sets
AEE	Aerobic endurance: minutes of work, rest 1–5 minutes
HT	Hypertrophy: 8–12 reps, relatively slow rate of movement
OC	Own choice

Gym program 1: gym test

Exercise	Results	Comments	Focus
Warmup Bike	5 minutes		
Warmup Paddle Machine	7 minutes		
Bench Press 1 RM		Max 5 sets allowed	Maximum strength
Bench Pull 1 RM		Max 5 sets allowed Max 5 cm bench	Maximum strength
Bench Press 2 minutes 55 kg			Strength endurance
Bench Pull 2 minutes 55 kg		Max 5 cm bench	Strength endurance
Chins 1 RM		Max allowed 80 kg; more than this and the athlete should do reps	Maximum strength
Dips 1 RM		Max allowed 80 kg; more than this and the athlete should do reps	Maximum strength
Chins Max Reps			Strength endurance
Dips Max Reps			Strength endurance
Stretching on Completion			Flexibility

Gym program 2

Exercise	Sets*reps	Comments	Focus
Warmup Paddle Machine	7 minutes		
Circuit (Dumbbell Curls, Dumbbell Bench Pulls, Dumbbell Bench Press)	2[3*18–25)]	One set is the three exercises done three times each with no rest.	Endurance and lactate tolerance
Circuit (Dips, Chins, Incline Abs)	2[3*18–25)]	One set is the three exercises done three times each with no rest.	Endurance and lactate tolerance
Circuit (Lat Pulldowns, Tricep Extension, Single Dumbbell Pulls)	2[3*18–25)]	One set is the three exercises done three times each with no rest.	Endurance and lactate tolerance
Abs	200		Stabilization
Warm-Down Paddle Machine/On Water	10 minutes		Technique

Gym program 3

Exercise	Sets*reps	Comments	Focus
Warmup Paddle Machine	7 minutes		
Dumbbell Bench Press	4*2–6		Max strength
Dumbbell Bench Pull	4*2–6		Max strength
Dips	4*2–6		Max strength
Chins	4*2–6		Max strength
Bench Press	4*2–6		Max strength
Barbell Bench Pulls	4*2–6		Strength, coordination
Clean and Press	4*2–6		Strength, coordination
Abs	200		Stabilization
Warm-Down Paddle Machine/On Water	10 minutes		Technique

SECTION 2: SLALOM

Sylvain Curinier
Fédération Française de Canoë-Kayak (FFCK),
Joinville-le-Pont, France; INSEP, Paris, France;
and France PNL, Paris, France

The specificity of canoe/kayak slalom

In slalom, the way that paddlers express themselves on the course results in a mental and physical effort of about 100 seconds. The paddling type is special because it is completely acyclic, meaning that the nature of the effort will be fundamentally different compared to that of a straight-line race. Added to this, the canoe/kayak (CK) slalom playing field is the river, in the open. The goal, or "off plan," is to follow a set path through gates that take the form of two poles that must not be touched for fear of being given time penalties by the judges at the end of the race. The objective is to understand these elements as well as possible, in order to paddle with the greatest efficiency. *Great efficiency* means speed, accuracy, and ensuring that the fluctuations of the river have a minimal impact on the way that the paddlers express themselves and the final result. In my opinion, the best learning is task specific. The best training is, therefore, whitewater practice, on rivers that will reproduce all the characteristics of the major

event's competition course. The aim is for the progress to be continuous, permanent, and as quick as possible. This also means that the paddlers will need to be challenged by practice venues where they will be perpetually reassessing themselves, but that also contain a variety of difficulties. To date, even with modular artificial courses, it is essential to diversify the playing field in order to learn faster in different situations. By nature, slalom paddlers are nomadic adventurers who will express themselves better in novelty rather than in routine. It should be pointed out that even athletes who practice in a closed environment are training in diversified environments, because human nature needs change in order to be challenged and to progress faster. The thirst for understanding and for progression will be even greater with the desire and the joy of discovering new horizons. Muscular and physiological development is obviously interesting, but it is essential to combine it with other progression goals, especially the skill and precision required to navigate between poles, not to mention visual information retrieval and decision making.

Planning process: the META training

What is the planning process based on? See the five-branched star describing the META training in Figure 6.2.

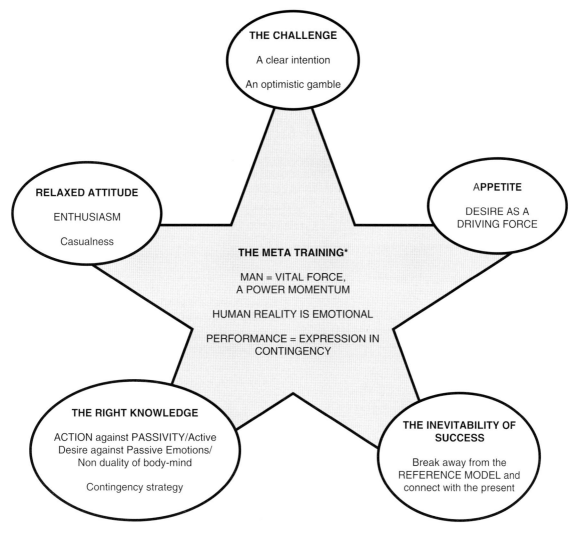

Figure 6.2 The five-branched star used in META training.

The basics of training

C/K slalom is the ultimate discipline where the athlete's success results from the combination of a multitude of dimensions of the human being. It is difficult and simplistic to define the many dimensions of the human being, but the main dimensions that are recognized in the world of sports are the physical dimension, the technical dimension, and the mental dimension.

My coaching style is very particular and can appear nonconforming. Indeed, my view of what constitutes the necessary preparation to win a World Championship or an Olympic gold medal does not match a "segmented" approach to training split between physical, technical, and mental preparation. Incidentally, I call it the META training (META comes from the Greek prefix meaning "after," "beyond," and "with"; it expresses everything at once: entirety, reflection, and change).

The concept of nonduality of body and mind

I distinguish between both the soul and the body as two separate things. Indeed, the experience of thinking, of the mind, is very different from that of the body. That said, the mind and the body are only two aspects of the same reality for me, two sides of the same coin. The mind and body cannot oppose each other, cannot contradict each other, cannot dissociate from one another. In short, training cannot be split between the mental and the physical and other dimensions. But how do we deal with this?

I understand that it is common to separate the mental, physical, and technical preparation; this is done out of convenience, but above all because it is the prevalent way of seeing things in sports and in the western world in which we evolve. In my case, I believe that the psychological aspect of each individual is closely linked to their body, the way they use it, and the way it develops. The more the body is understood, its needs respected, and its flaws and fragility accepted, the more it welcomes desire and pleasure, and the more it progresses. This is why it is crucial to rely on the methods of physical training, mental training, and technical training that successfully include all of these aspects.

In my view, when the wrong paradigm is used to address a training that has to make sense for the athletes who we coach, we are on the wrong track. This can cause great disappointment and unsolvable problems when faced with the inevitable failures that occur in high-level sports. In my opinion, segmented or categorized training is a misrepresentation of the world, a line of thought that seems easier to follow at first, but that ultimately turns out to be inconsistent with my views on the human condition. In this epistemological framework, I rely on a symbolism that I created with the athletes who I coach: the star of the META* training, which will systematically guide us in all our actions.

The definition of performance for inevitable success

For me, this includes the following questions: how do I conceptualize performance, and what is my representation of the human condition in all this? These are epistemological and philosophical discussions, and I will try to explain myself on the subject.

I believe that human reality is primarily an emotional reality. The body and mind cannot be separated. Basically, we are primarily a desire to live, a desire to be, and a desire to preserve and enhance what we are. It is from our emotions, our joys, our fears, our moods, and our passions that our life comes together, and that the Olympic gold medal is won. Our preparation is built upon this emotional jungle, and the performance takes place in these "unfathomable depths." Without desire, there is no action, no initiative – in short, no life. And it is therefore crucial to recognize that the notion of desire, accompanied by the pleasure to express ourselves, overrides the notion of will. This is what I try to apply during each training session. To prepare for a competition to that end is much more important than to train. To prepare for the inevitability of success is to wish to embrace fully and without any compromise the desire to grow, to be assertive and to perform, to increase one's power, life force, through the traps, obstacles, but also the opportunities presented to us. The competition will thus be understood as a place of expression, among many others, available to the athletes.

Understand and accept the situation of competition/accept the idea of contingency

The competitive situation is complex and especially contingent. If we want everyone to be able to express themselves in a contingent competition situation, we must adopt a proper strategy and mindset. What is contingency?

Contingency is the idea that we cannot predict the future, which is by definition uncertain, unpredictable, and completely unknown. The unknown is the essence of the competitive situation, especially as the playing or expression field of the competitors is located on a river made of incessant fluctuations and the uncertainties of complex water movements. The strategy of contingency thus consists in using daily the uncertain situations, randomness, and the indeterminate to one's advantage. This strategy is key to the training model. By definition, the river and the white-water generate incredibly complex fluctuations and uncertainties. They have to be used as well as possible by the paddler, whose ultimate goal is to realize its full potential in the allotted time. Along the way, the paddler will evolve toward a more adequate understanding of the situation. The definition of the strategy is obviously to leave the pre-established program, but more so, to immerse ourselves in a certain context in order to move forward with optimism and determination in a constant search for progress and joy to navigate. For joy is, in my eyes, the only way to learn properly. What is learning and progressing appropriately? In fact, the experience of knowledge is more important than the stock of knowledge itself. The division of training into physical, technical, and mental preparation has its limitations and can ultimately lead athletes to hit a wall. Remember that, for me, a human's growth to being whole has almost no limit. However, using this type of training successfully is quite an art. Significant resources are to be implemented for this type of training, as well as the necessity to be surrounded by trustworthy people, expert in their field of intervention. They must display strong ethical attitudes and use the specific tools of the META training (physical therapist, yoga instructor, optometrist, coach action type approach, aroma-therapy, and symbolic modeling therapist).

This strategy is based on the following question: how can we learn to cope with uncertainty and emerge from it stronger than before? In my eyes, it is a priority for sports training, which can be extended to each and every person's life. For the essential question that every CK slalom paddler faces is: "How do I successfully be the best, despite the vagaries of the river that may greatly influence the level of difficulty of a figure, or the arrival time?" To do this, we have to learn how to "paddle on a river of uncertainties thanks to a certainty support." This support will be directly linked to the way the paddler expresses him or herself on the water:

1 His propulsion efficiency
2 His balancing skills

3 His visual perception in order to move through the poles and manage his trajectories.

To do so, a series of three to four workouts on these aspects is necessary. Since the body and mind have their own limits, it is important to plan the sessions in advance and to adapt them in order to obtain a significant level of quality and, above all, a positive and constructive experience for the athletes. They are the ones who will set their own limits on this matter, along with the coach.

What kind of training? 75% technical! "Paddling on a river of uncertainties, thanks to a certainty support"

Many workouts are called *technical*. They vary in their form, adapt to particular contexts, and are always guided by a sense of play, novelty, efficiency of navigation, and pleasure to progress.

Reminder: The various certainty supports will be linked to the paddler's characteristic style, not to the external context:

1 Propulsion efficiency
2 Balancing skills
3 Visual perception in order to move through the poles and manage the trajectories.

Canoeing technique

Technique represents the largest volume of training. In terms of training sessions, it represents approximately two workouts out of three. The technique can be broken down in terms of objectives and progress:

• The *navigation skills*: Balance, ease, and accuracy in the overcoming and handling of different movements of water (falls, deflectors, waves, rollers, countercurrents, etc.)

• The *effectiveness* (the speed–precision pair) of different trajectories through the gates (upstream gates, staggered downstream gates), and of the different approaches to technical negotiating of the poles (stops, zigzag, reversal, dodging, etc.)

• Also, the *efficiency* of the supports' transmission and the use of the boat's qualities in order to turn, accelerate, or slow down.

Thanks to the lifting up of the boats, facilitated by a conveyor belt in artificial rivers, the number of descents has increased during a practice time that is often limited to 60 minutes (due to the allotted navigation slots). It is important not to cool down too much between each session and thus to reduce the time spent on the analysis that will be done afterward, for each workout is filmed so as to make an analysis video of the different turns. The goal is to keep learning "on the ground," to develop an understanding of what is happening on the river and between the gates. Indeed, during live training, there is too much information to be considered simultaneously. This is when the intuitive and experienced eye of the coach can become an asset, along with the insight of very experienced athletes, allowing them to progress faster.

The desire to progress faster: the will to master skills that will not be shaken during highly emotional situations such as competition

As can be understood, I believe that the physical and muscular approach does not appear to determine success in CK slalom and even proves inadequate compared to a more comprehensive approach. The training of different physical and physiological qualities will therefore always be done with larger objectives in mind. The progression in terms of the physical dimension will thus always be useful for technical skills and navigation. It is also used to improve the capacity of the paddler to navigate more efficiently and longer on challenging rivers and courses in order to learn better and faster. This is because, in my eyes, the time spent desiring to navigate more efficiently is what makes the difference. It is not normal to be constantly tired and to have no desire to always improve when navigating. Unfortunately, too many paddlers do so. As far

as I am concerned, the word *work* is prohibited during training – because I do not think that "work" generates medals. Athletes do not deserve their medals simply because they work well and a lot. On the contrary, they deserve it if they manage to maintain their own joy to make further progress every day and to exceed their own limits.

Aerobic and anaerobic capacity

Basic aerobics is best executed out of the slalom boat (usually some footing, cycling, or, more rarely, cross-country skiing), once a week.

The goal is to navigate at racing speed, hence the large number of sessions divided by rounds of five to eight gates, which correspond to anaerobic capacities.

Specific aerobics takes the form of "loops," allowing the athlete to cover kilometers of highly technical rivers, but limiting the difficulty of the trajectories, and thus limiting the number of gates on the course. In general, they are programmed two to three times per week.

An example of specific aerobic training: three sets of three descents, 1 min 30 to 2 minutes in whitewater + 1 minute in flat water (1 min 30 in conveyor belt lifts). The course is either imposed or improvised with a maximum of four upstream gates.

Split shifts with flat-water gates negotiating are programmed in order to increase power in preparation for the training set dedicated to the specific competition effort. Two sets (10 minutes) 6 × 25 (a judged and timed course downstream to 4–5 gates, with relaxed paddling back upstream) are recommended.

Training intensities

Many racing-speed sessions are between 15 and 25 seconds, which allows keeping a perceptive focus and navigating to competition speed.

Strength training

Strength and specific power training is fundamental. However, this type of training is preceded by a diagnosis of primary reflexes and by specific integration work. The goal is to stabilize the new skills on driving foundations that will not be shaken by the emotional charge of the competition.

During winter training: two to three times a week; during competition training: once a week+some warmups.

• These sessions are carried out of the boat, standing on one or two feet with movement of the arms slowed down and disturbed by an elastic band. This originated from a physiotherapeutic approach for the prevention and strengthening of structural deep muscles of the spine and shoulders. I have "hijacked" it to create real muscle-strengthening sessions whose objective is fourfold:

1 Movements that are always from the proximal to the distal (from the center of gravity toward the fingers, head, and feet). The movements organized around the elastic band allow the athlete to mimic the natural expression of the paddle stroke by "creating support in water" in a situation of instability.

2 The idea is to combine, solicit, and thus simultaneously enhance the qualities of balance, coordination, speed, strength, and endurance.

3 Has the benefit of improving strength, speed, and endurance, without suffering technical loss in the boat

4 Guarantees the prevention of injuries to the shoulders and spine throughout the season.

• The core stabilizing and building of the deep muscles of the spine (transverse, perineum) in the form of rather isokinetic endurance postures during 3–4 minutes

• Isokinetic strengthening on machines such as the Biodex or Contrex in order to push the limits and progress in speed creation on each support. An isokinetic set on the depressors and rotators. A set spread over 3 weeks of around eight sessions, 12 weeks before the first season goal. It is possible to recall this type of training just after the first

deadline of the season, if the second season is happening 4 months after.

• Loops aerobic sessions at below-maximum speed in the boat, slowing down during winter.

• Isokinetic sessions on specific gestures (circular supports in kayak and cross draw in canoe) following the technical set of winter preparation.

Optometry

A visual workout session is scheduled almost every week to develop various visual qualities (focalization, focalization endurance, etc.).

Kinesiotherapy, osteopathy, and aromatherapy

It is essential to combine this type of training sessions with recovery and prevention sessions (osteopathy and kinesiotherapy, acupuncture, and aromatherapy) taught by professionals abiding by the META* training.

Designing the full training program

Yearly plan

Example: Figure 6.3 – Tony Estanguet's 2012 program document.

The yearly plan consists of two main periods. The first one aims to prepare for the national team selections; it has a 7-month duration between October and April. The second is shorter and ends with the World Championships or the Olympics; it lasts for approximately 4 months, between May and September. Each period is composed of blocs with a specific dominant.

For all periods, the goal is to paddle on as many international-level whitewater courses as possible.

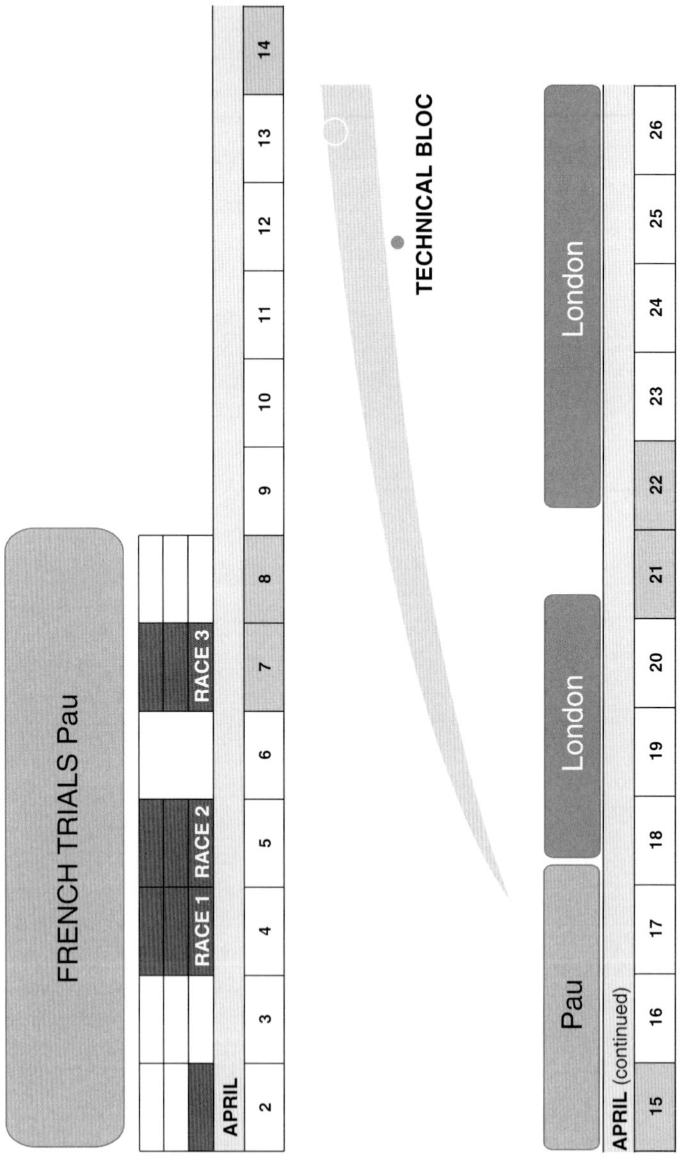

Figure 6.3 Tony Estanguet: 2012 program.

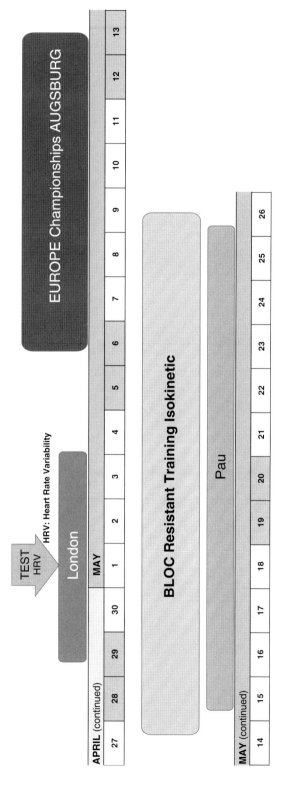

Figure 6.3 *(Continued)*

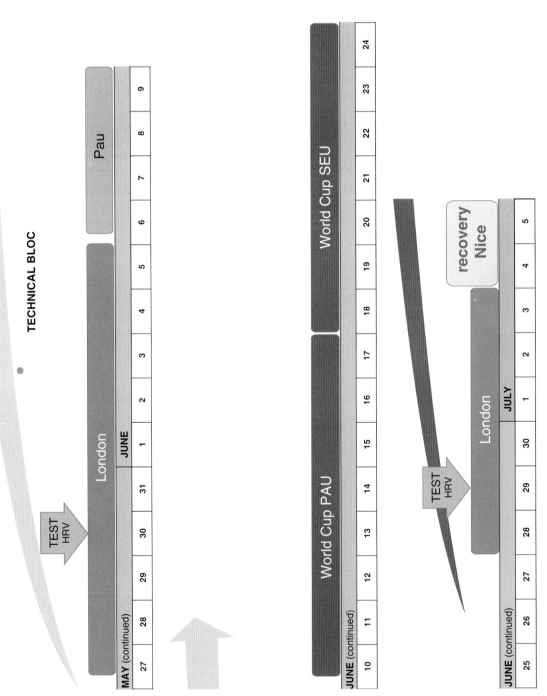

Figure 6.3 (*Continued*)

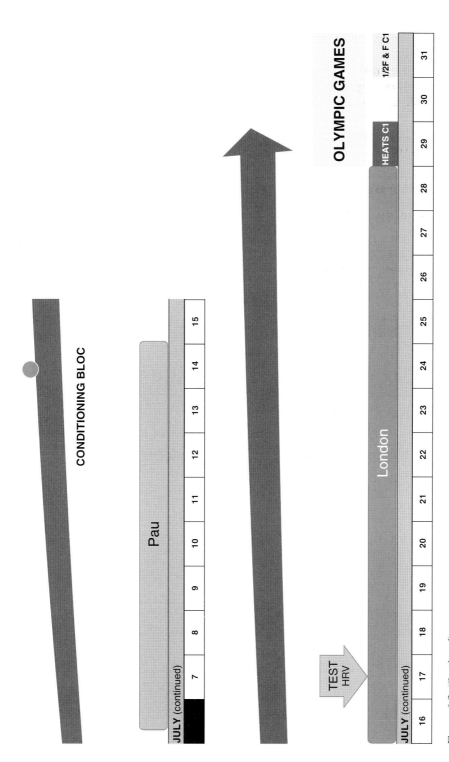

Figure 6.3 *(Continued)*

- Period 1: October to April
  - Technical development bloc: 6 weeks in October–November
  - Isokinetic bloc resistance training: 4 weeks in November–December
  - Break + aerobic development bloc: end of the year, 2 weeks in late December–early January (skiing, etc.)
  - Winter technical development bloc: 4 weeks, Australia
  - Pre-competition bloc: 6 weeks
  - Tapering bloc: 2 weeks

- Period 2
  - 5 weeks: First international competitions period and specific training on Olympic slalom course
  - 2 weeks: Isokinetic sessions on specific gestures
  - 2 weeks: Technical set
  - 2 weeks: Competition training, World Cup series
  - 5 weeks: Reviewing

Designing a weekly training program

Example: Pre-competition bloc (D-3 weeks)

BLOC 1 prépa Piges							
Tuesday	**Wednesday**	**Thursday**	**Friday**	**Saturday**	**Sunday**	**Monday**	**Tuesday**
6	7	8	9	10	11	12	13
RM gainage	Tech tiers	RM	Tech	Longs	RM	Longs	RM
Loops I2	I3 30″30″	Tech	Quarts/demis		LIBRE	I3 30″30″	Loops I2
Tech		Loops I3				I1	Tech libre

Gainage: Postural muscle building. I1: Low-intensity aerobic. I3: High-intensity aerobic. LIBRE: Free to decide what to do is the best for progress. Longs: Like race design 100 seconds. Loops I2: Loops, medium-intensity aerobic. Loops I3: Loops, high-intensity aerobic. Quarts/demis: 1/2 course. On each half, two different sections of 5–6 gates. RM: Resistance training. Tech: Technical.

Bibliography

Bishop, D. (2000). Physiological predictors of flat-water kayak performance in women. *Eur J Appl Physiol* 82 (1–2): 91–97.

Bonetti, D.L. and Hopkins, W.G. (2010). Variation in performance times of elite flat-water canoeists from race to race. *Int J Sports Physiol Perform* 5 (2): 210–217.

Jackson, P.S., Locke, N., and Brown, P. (1992) The hydrodynamics of paddle propulsion. Paper presented at the 11th Australian Fluid Mechanics Conference, University of Tasmania, Hobart, Australia.

Michael, J., Smith, R., and Rooney, K. (2009). Determinants of kayak paddling performance. *Sports Biomechanics* 8 (2): 167–179.

Svenska Kanotförbundet [Sweden Canoe and Kayak Federation]. (2009) SKF:s Kravanalys Kajak Sprint. Ursviken, Sweden: Svenska Kanotförbundet.

Chapter 7
Medical problems in canoeing and kayaking

Bo Berglund

Department of Medicine, Karolinska University Hospital, Solna, Sweden

Training and competing at the elite level place a great deal of stress on the individual. Paddlers, especially elite paddlers, therefore face many of the usual problems seen in sports medicine.

Environmental factors

The specific medical problems of canoeing are often related to environmental factors in connection with accidental turn-overs during training or competition. Many elite paddlers strive to train year-round on the water. During the winter, the water is colder, and there is an increased risk of softening of the skin or trenchfoot, as well as of hypothermia and drowning if the paddler should fall into the water. A sudden immersion can cause hyperventilation, bronchospasm, and cardiac arrest due to the shock of cold water. Longer exposure results in skeletal muscle weakness, loss of capability to maintain thermoregulation, and development of hypothermia.

Therefore, when the water is cold, all paddlers are advised to wear adequate clothing (such as splash-covers and wetsuits) and flotation devices (such as a lifejacket), and to ensure that their boats have enough buoyant support. Although drowning is uncommon among elite paddlers, it must be given serious consideration as a risk when training on cold water. A good method is to teach young paddlers that "there are equal amounts of water close to the shore as in the middle of the lake."

Heat produced during exercise in a hot, humid environment cannot be readily dissipated from the body. Therefore, during prolonged exercise in the heat, there is a risk of developing fatigue secondary to hyperthermia. When accompanied by dehydration, heat exhaustion may lead to hypovolemia, an inability to provide both skeletal muscle and skin with oxygenated blood in required rates, and heat stroke, a potentially lethal disorder characterized by disturbed consciousness and organ damage.

Another common environmental problem is solar radiation. During the summer months, there is a considerable risk for sun-related medical problems due to increased exposure, diminished ozone levels, and additional reflections from the water. Sunburn is a common problem, and other solar-induced diseases such as melanomas are increasing in frequency, particularly in the fair-skinned population. Paddlers are prone to the development of pterygium, a growth of the connective tissue that can extend over the conjunctiva. This ophthalmological condition is promoted by exposure to wind, water, and sun. Several cases of this condition have been reported in paddlers, and excision of the lesion is necessary. Therefore, it is recommended that all paddlers wear sun protection (such as protective clothes, hats, sunscreens, and sunglasses).

Some diseases responsible for turn-overs

Most turn-overs in elite paddlers are accidental, but it is important to diagnose and treat disorders that can cause transient unconsciousness or an inability to maintain balance. It must be realized that these diseases are not dangerous per se, but may be hazardous due to the fact that they may lead to turn-overs. Most elite paddlers are young and healthy, but despite an excellent profile, they may have such underlying diseases. Many uncommon, mostly genetic diseases may cause unconsciousness, but they will not be discussed here.

Neurological diseases

Exercise-induced syncope is a fairly common problem. It is the result of global cerebral ischemia due to failure of cerebral perfusion. Perfusion failure during, or shortly after, a prolonged exertion, such as hard endurance training, may be related to cutaneous vasodilation while muscle blood vessels are still dilated, compromising cardiac output and resulting in syncope. Migraine attacks (effort migraine) can occur after athletic effort of any kind. Many effort migraine attacks have only parts of the classic migraine. Severe headache, scotomas, occasional hyperventilation, and nausea usually occur immediately after exertion. Focal neurological deficits are seldom seen. The symptoms may be precipitated by dehydration, excessive heat, hypoglycemia, and unaccustomed altitude. Effort migraine is more common in untrained athletes, and it tends to decrease provided that physical fitness improves and other precipitating factors are avoided.

Cardiac disease and sudden death (SD)

Paroxysmal atrial tachycardia (PAT) is a common type of cardiac arrhythmia seen in young athletes. It is usually a benign re-entry arrhythmia with a duration of seconds to hours. During the attacks of tachycardia, the cardiac output decreases, and symptoms such as dizziness and syncope may occur. PAT can be precipitated by dehydration, hypoglycemia, and drugs like beta-stimulators and caffeine. This arrhythmia often diminishes with increasing age and the absence of precipitating factors. PAT can be treated successfully with pharmacological agents, but several of these medications (especially beta-blockers) decrease exercise capacity as well.

Wolf–Parkinson–White (WPW) syndrome occurs due to the presence of a congenital anomalous atrioventricular conduction pathway. WPW syndrome is associated with attacks of tachycardia, sometimes very fast and of long duration. These attacks decrease cardiac output, and symptoms such as dizziness and syncope may occur. At present, WPW syndrome can be treated successfully by pharmacological and surgical methods.

SD in young adults and young athletes is uncommon: SD's incidence is around 1 per 100 000 people per year. Underlying cardiac disease is the most common cause of SD. The most common cardiac causes include electrical abnormalities within a structurally normal heart, and different types of cardiomyopathies, including hypertrophic cardiomyopathy (HCM). In athletes older than 35, the major cause of SD is coronary atherosclerosis.

HCM is a congenital disease and a common cause of SD (more so during exercise) due to malignant ventricular arrhythmias in young athletes. The symptoms are often few and may include accentuated dyspnea, dizziness, and syncope. The disease is a contraindication for exertional sports and training, including canoeing and kayaking. HCM often causes echocardiography (EchoCG) abnormalities and is diagnosed with EchoCG.

Endocrine disease

Type 1 diabetes mellitus is insulin dependent, and most often young individuals are affected. With proper insulin treatment, many diabetic patients can participate on a high athletic level (including the Olympics). Glycemic control is, however, extremely important in paddlers, since both hypo- and hyperglycemia may lead to disturbed consciousness.

Respiratory diseases

Exercise-induced asthma (EIA) is common in the athletic population. EIA that occurs on the water, however, may cause balance problems for the paddler, especially if the EIA is severe and/or the paddler has difficulty finding the inhalers (see below).

Exercise-induced asthma

EIA is used to describe symptoms of asthma, such as cough, wheeze, or dyspnea, provoked by vigorous physical activity.

High prevalence rates have been reported in athletes, and the type of activity (higher in endurance-type sports) and/or training conditions (higher in winter sports) influence the prevalence of asthma. Approximately 10% of Olympic summer athletes have EIA.

There is evidence that high-level, long-term endurance training may influence not only airway function but also structure. Environmental exposure, mechanical stress to the airways, frequent respiratory infections, and dysautonomia all contribute to the development of EIA. They cause airway inflammation and structural changes (remodeling), and variable airway obstruction. Fortunately, these changes may be partly reversible after cessation of training.

As canoeists have high levels of ventilation during intense exercise, exposure to cold air and environmental air contaminants such as allergens and pollutants is increased as compared to other sports.

Few studies have examined the optimal management of asthma in the athlete; it is currently recommended that asthma in the canoeist should be managed according to current national and international guidelines. The goals of asthma management are similar to those of the non-athlete: to minimize symptoms and optimize pulmonary function. They also help maximize sport performances, particularly in preventing EIA and comorbid conditions frequently observed in athletes, such as upper respiratory infection (URI), which may affect asthma control and should be identified and treated.

Diagnosis and pharmacological management must be carefully performed, with particular consideration of current antidoping regulations, when caring for athletes. Based on the demonstration that the inhaled asthma drugs do not improve performance in healthy athletes, the doping regulations are presently much less strict than previously. It is considered very important for asthmatic individuals to master EIA to be able to participate in physical activity on an equal level with their peers, and a precise early diagnosis with optimal treatment follow-up is vital in this aspect.

Nonpharmacological measures

Asthma education is considered an essential component of asthma management. Monitoring of asthma control criteria, preventative measures, and management of exacerbations should be part of acquired self-management skills.

For the canoeist, allergens present in the training environment should be identified, although it is often difficult to avoid such exposure. Emotions and stress may worsen asthma symptoms, but good asthma control may help reduce their effects.

A low-intensity exercise (warm-up) before exertion may induce a "refractory period" to exercise for a period of about two hours. Whenever possible, athletes should avoid training when air quality is poor or in extreme conditions of temperature and humidity. Mechanical barriers, such as face masks, may counteract the effects of cold air or some pollutants, but they are often not tolerated due to the high ventilation required during exercise.

Pharmacological treatment

Asthma pharmacotherapy in the canoeist should be individualized and based on the reduction of inflammation, mainly with inhaled corticosteroids (ICSs). ICSs can reduce EIA in most patients after a few weeks of regular use. Rapid-acting beta$_2$-agonists are the most frequently used "reliever" medications for intermittent symptoms and prevention of EIA. Protection against EIB diminishes, however, when these agents are used regularly, and they should therefore be used at the minimum dose and frequency required to minimize this loss of effect.

If asthma is not controlled by a low dose of ICS, current guidelines suggest that long-acting beta$_2$-agonists (LABAs) should be prescribed to improve such control, while leukotriene antagonists are a second-choice option for this purpose. Monotherapy with LABAs should not be allowed, as it may be associated with a worsening of asthma and severe asthma events. Oral corticosteroids may be needed for severe asthma exacerbations, but these may require a therapeutic use exemption (TUE). All athletes must comply with World Anti-Doping Agency (WADA) regulations for the use of asthma medications.

Inhaled beta$_2$-agonists are the best preventative medication for EIA and, when used before exercise (e.g. 10–15 minutes), may reduce airway response to exercise.

Medical problems associated with sympathetic nervous activity and adaptation to intense training in elite athletes

The sympathetic nervous system is of utmost importance for the adaptation of the body to physical exercise (i.e. the training effect). The sympathetic nervous system uses catecholamines (adrenaline and noradrenaline) to elicit its effects. The adrenaline present in the blood originates from sympathetic stimulation of the adrenal medulla, and this secretion sustains the action of the sympathetic nerves. By contrast, most of the plasma noradrenaline is due to overflow from the sympathetic nerve endings.

All athletic activities require voluntary motor recruitment, but feedback from skeletal muscle afferents plays an essential role in regulating sympathetic nervous system outflow as well as blood pressure, augmentation in cardiac output, and the distribution of skeletal muscle blood flow.

The sympathetic nervous system outflow may, however, also contribute to some medical problems associated with maladaptation and excessive release of catecholamine in elite endurance athletes.

Physical training induces adaptation to the sympathetic nervous system. Although the 24 hour average adrenaline and noradrenaline concentrations are twice as high in trained as compared to untrained subjects, endurance training in general results in a lower plasma adrenaline concentration at any given absolute workload. However, when compared at identical relative workloads as well as in response to numerous non-exercise stimuli, trained endurance athletes have a higher catecholamine secretion capacity compared to sedentary individuals.

Catecholamine concentration is more affected by intensity than duration of physical exercise, and the sympathetic nervous system is more activated in high-intensity than endurance-trained athletes. There is also a marked increase in catecholamine concentration above lactate threshold and maximal oxygen uptake (VO_{2max}), especially so for higher intensities, and after a second daily training bout. Thus, the basal catecholamine concentration, according to studies, can be multiplied by 5–10 times and occasionally even more at exercises up to 160% of VO_{2max}. The same increase in catecholamine has, however, been noted also after long-distance (50 km) cross-country skiing competition in world-class endurance athletes. Furthermore, long-term endurance exercise also is able to induce, for several hours, a sustained sympathetic activation after exercise.

The effect of exercise training on sympathetic nerve responses per se is complex. But one interesting effect with endurance training is a blunted chronotropic – and augmented inotropic – response to the sympathetic nerve activity of the heart. This blunting of chronotropic activity also can be noted during acute long-term (24 hours) exercise tests at essentially constant load. The underlying mechanism behind the decrease in heart rate is most likely a beta-receptor downregulation and/or desensitization.

Sympathetic nervous system outflow and adrenal endocrine capacity can be limiting factors for performance in world-class endurance athletes. Overtraining, increased risk of infections, and abnormal heart function in connection with long-term exercise are known consequences of maladaptation to exercise in elite endurance athletes.

When excessive training stress is applied concurrent with inadequate recovery, performance decrements and maladaptation may occur. Known as the *overtraining syndrome*, this complex condition can afflict endurance athletes. The importance of the sympathetic nervous system for adaptation of training stress is supported by controlled studies, where this syndrome is associated with burnout and at least a 50% decrease in basal catecholamine excretion, thus indicating downregulation or inadequate secretion/sympathetic nervous outflow.

Alterations in mucosal immunity are also related to the activation of the sympathetic nervous system. The production of secretory immunoglobulin-A (IgA) provides the "first line of defense" against upper respiratory tract (URT) pathogens. Prolonged exercise and intensified training can decrease saliva secretion of IgA, and consensus exists that reduced levels of saliva IgA are associated with increased risk of URT infections (Walsh et al. 2011). Mechanisms underlying this decreased immunity are related to the activation of the sympathetic nervous system and its associated effects.

The idea that cardiac injury could develop from physical activity was first suggested at the end of the twentieth century. The most likely mechanism for cardiac injury is an excessive release of catecholamine, which may result in catecholamine-related toxic effects on the heart, including substantial structural alterations, which seem to have a pivotal role in the development of stress cardiomyopathy (also called Takutsobu cardiomyopathy) or high-output heart failure. These conditions have been described in ultra-endurance athletes and after long-distance Ironman triathlons. It is possible that this finding is of clinical importance, since swimmers and triathletes may develop so-called swimming pulmonary edema, which in some cases can be lethal. However, transient pulmonary edema also has been found in other endurance athletes, such as elite cyclists (McKenzie et al. 2005). Therefore, due to their transient nature, it is most likely that catecholamine-related effects on the heart are underdiagnosed in elite endurance athletes.

Specific medical problems for female paddlers

Female elite paddlers have the same medical problems as male paddlers. There are, however, a few additional problems that must be stressed. As in other endurance sports, the hard training necessary for world-class paddlers may lead to disturbed menstruation and amenorrhea (see Chapter 3). Female athletes also have a lower intake and larger losses of iron than do male athletes, and therefore female athletes run an increased risk of developing a hypochromic anemia that may decrease their performance. Iron deficiency is most easily diagnosed by hemoglobin concentration and serum ferritin (an indicator of iron stores). Regular checkups are recommended. It must, however, be emphasized that iron supplements will enhance performance in individuals who have iron-deficiency anemia, but not in athletes with normal iron stores.

Preparticipation screening

Preparticipation screening of canoeists is therefore recommended and should consist of a medical history questionnaire, a physical examination, and physiological tests such as ECG. A positive family history and/or cardiovascular symptoms such as chest pain, dyspnea, dizziness and syncope, and/or abnormal ECG should be followed by an extended health evaluation, including ECG. Blood and urine tests to determine hemoglobin and iron status, or to detect unsuspected disease, are done routinely in many countries. Specific attention should be paid to the musculoskeletal system of these athletes. A detailed history and physical examination of the shoulders are necessary to access range of motion, strength, and muscular imbalance. If it is available, objective measurements of the strength of the internal and external rotators of the shoulder also should be done.

Anti-doping

Canoe and kayak races in the Olympic Games have a duration from approximately 30 seconds to 4 minutes, whereas, in addition, at World Championships there also are longer marathon events with a duration of up to several hours. Elite paddlers therefore need high aerobic and anaerobic capacity and also a high maximal power. Doping agents or methods improving these capacities may also improve paddling performance, and the use of such substances and methods in paddlers was comprehensive in some countries (Berendonk 1991). As a result of these findings, the International Canoe Federation (ICF) took early and firm action against doping and started comprehensive out-of-competition testing of elite paddlers.

ICF has been a stakeholder of WADA from the start and today follows the rules and regulations of the WADA Code. The WADA Code applies to all national- or international-level athletes, and they are defined by the National Anti-Doping Organization or ICF, respectively. If an athlete is merely engaged in recreational activities, National Anti-Doping Organizations also have the discretion to decide whether and how the Code will apply. The roles and responsibilities of athletes are included in the WADA Code. WADA keeps a list of substances and methods that at a given moment are banned; for more information, see the WADA website (www.wada-ama.org).

ICF has also started an anti-doping education program called Pure Paddling Performance, which preserves the "spirit of sport" by educating all canoeing athletes and team support personnel on the issue of anti-doping. On completing the program, athletes will know more about health risks and their rights and responsibilities regarding anti-doping. Pure Paddling Performance provides an interactive learning experience made up of interactive videos and questions on a range of topics, including testing, TUEs, and whereabouts. The program is now available in five languages.

Bibliography

Baker, S. and Atha, J. (1981). Canoeist's disorientation following cold water immersion. *Br J Sports Med* 5: 111–115.

Berendonk, B. (1991). *Doping dokumente. Von der Forschung zum Betrug.* Berlin: Springer Verlag.

Del Giacco, S.R., Firinu, D., Bjermer, L., and Carlsen, K.H. (2015). Exercise and asthma: an overview. *Eur Clin Respir J* 2: 279–284.

Maron, B.J. and Pelliccia, A. (2006). The heart of trained athletes: cardiac remodeling and the risks of sports, including sudden death. *Circulation* 114: 1633–1644.

McKenzie, D.C., O'Hare, T.J., and Mayo, J. (2005). The effect of sustained heavy exercise on the development of pulmonary edema in trained male cyclists. *Respir Physiol Neurobiol* 145: 209–218.

Walsh, N.P., Gleeson, M., Shephard, R.J. et al. (2011). Position statement. Part one: immune function and exercise. *Exerc Immunol Rev* 17: 6–63.

Chapter 8
Orthopaedic injuries in canoeing

Jozsef Dobos

Department of Sport Surgery, National Institute of Sports Medicine, Budapest, Hungary

Introduction

Canoeing has several disciplines – flatwater (or sprint), slalom, canoe sailing, ocean racing, dragon boat, marathon, wildwater, canoe polo, freestyle, and standup paddleboarding – which have been expanding rapidly in the last decade. Sprint and slalom are in the program of the Olympic Games. Although canoeing is widespread, the number of published scientific studies concerning injuries in the sport is regrettably low. In several existing studies, data of professional and free-time athletes, comprising junior, adult, and senior sportsmen, are combined. The majority of the studies cover recreational and competitive wildwater racing, as there are more injuries and dangers in this discipline (e.g. hypothermia following turn-over). Authors of some studies only analyze disorders of specific parts of the body – wrist, lumbar spine, shoulder, and so on – or report on one discipline exclusively. There are a few general studies covering several disciplines; however, there is not a single sourcebook covering elite flatwater and slalom paddlers, reporting on a high number of cases with long follow-up, that is known to this author. My experiences in this field have been summarized, and I believe the incidence of injuries is relevant.

General characteristics of canoeing and kayaking

Canoeing and kayaking are sports with cyclical and relatively low-intensity movement. *Low intensity* means that the athlete produces only a force not higher than 20–25 kpa. Water is a soft medium; therefore, at the start of paddling, there is no need for extremely high intensity. However, the frequency and speed of this movement are high, and a successful competitor has to maintain a very high stroke rate for as long as possible. Paddling requires a delicate blend of power and endurance.

There is no body contact and no weightbearing on the legs, but the movements in canoeing have to be performed in an extremely unstable position. Balance problems can be caused by wind, wind-generated waves, and turbulence. New manufacturing techniques have increased instability in kayaks and canoes; they are becoming narrower. The synchrony of activity of different muscle groups can be disturbed by abrupt movements of the arms and body trying to preserve stability. This may result in muscle injuries of the trunk. The soft medium, water, makes start easier but makes supporting more difficult.

Canoeing is an open-air sport. Canoeing can take place in extremely high temperatures, and the

Canoeing, First Edition. Edited by Don McKenzie and Bo Berglund.
© 2019 International Olympic Committee. Published 2019 by John Wiley & Sons Ltd.

competitors are exposed to direct and indirect sunlight, reflected by water. Athletes involved in strenuous exercise in the heat and humidity may lose a lot of water and electrolytes. This electrolyte imbalance may result in reduced muscle contractility, and it is the next cause of muscle injuries. Kayakers can also be exposed to environmental pollution. The medical effect of this is several skin infections (contact dermatitis) in the gluteal region, in the knee region, and on the hands.

Kayaking and canoeing are similar in physiological intensity but different for physical preparation and loading of the locomotor system. Kayaking needs symmetrical movements; the center of gravity is relatively low, the spinal column is loaded mainly by rotational movements, and injuries are common in the shoulder due to very long leverage.

In canoeing, loading is asymmetrical; the center of gravity is higher due to the kneeling position. Frequent, instinctive movements of the trunk are necessary to assure stability. Flexion and extension are significant in the spinal column, and potential damage to the knee is a risk.

Clinical biomechanics

Outstanding studies are available analyzing movements of the trunk, the shoulder region, the pelvis, the knee joint, and the loading. The movements of kayaking and canoeing will only be described in general.

Kayaking

In the kayak stroke, the competitor has to make intense muscle contraction at the "catch" (when the paddle touches the water) because the boat accelerates and the resistance of the water decreases. The movement is described as pulling, but the motion is primarily in the trunk muscles as the competitor "leans down" the blade and attempts to move the boat nearer the paddle while pulling. The longer the phase of pulling, the more economical the movement; that is why the competitor attempts to reach forward. On the spine and the pelvis, there are continuous pendulum-like rotational movements in a slightly hooked position. When the blade reaches the hip, the competitor lifts out the paddle (and a lot of water too) with his or her pulling arm. Then, a symmetrical phase of the movement begins on the other side. The blades of the paddle are not in a flat position, but nearly 90° rotated, so the competitor must twist it with his or her wrists. If the wrists break toward the dorsal or the palmar side during the phase of pulling, the extensor or flexor muscles are strained excessively; this can lead to epicondylitis, or tendosynovitis of the forearm.

Canoeing

Canoeing stroke technique is different. At the beginning of the cycle, the competitor's center of gravity is next to the edge of the boat. He supports on the blade and, using his core muscles, he pulls himself and the boat toward the paddle. The muscles of his arms, although they seem to pull, assist with stability. When putting the paddle in the water, the competitor pushes his body forward in about 40°. The lumbar lordosis increases, the kyphosis of the back decreases, and the spinal column is in a torsion of about 30°. The competitor leans his body on the blade; therefore, at the side of the pulling hand, the back is concave. On the lumbar part of the spinal column, a convex scoliosis develops. At the side of the pulling arm, the back and abdominal muscles produce a larger force than at the side of the top hand. In the course of pulling, when the speed of the boat increases, the muscle tension decreases. The torsion and flexion of the spinal column diminish, the tension of the body muscles of the other side grows, but the predominance of the muscles at the side of the pulling arm remains the same. When the competitor lifts the paddle out of the water, his trunk is in a contralateral torsion of about 10°. After this, the paddle is thrust forward again, and the cycle is repeated. Most of the work is done by the back and shoulder muscles; most of the power is generated by the rotating body muscles. As the blade of the paddle is flat, no water is lifted out, and that is why loading of the muscles of the shoulder region is less than that of the kayakers. Because a canoe does not have a rudder, the athlete must steer the boat with both hands by flexing his wrists.

The canoe can cover a distance of 5–7 m at a stroke. The frequency of paddling is 35–40 per minute. Competitors cover more than 3000 km a year, so they perform the movement described here more than half a million times a year.

Performance

The steady improvement in performance in professional sport is particularly impressive in canoeing. This statement is illustrated by Table 8.1. The performance increases seen over a 20-year period have been measured by comparing the results achieved by Olympic champions. Track-and-field and swimming events have been chosen as benchmarks, as they are of similar duration and have comparable physiological demands. The changes in results over the 20-year period preceding the period under examination have been recorded. All comparisons show the progress of kayaking as the most dynamic (Table 8.1), partly owing to improved biomechanics and physical training adaptations. The development of equipment also played a vital role, although these changes were most important in the period between 1984 and 2004, when the new type of paddles and standards of boat building were introduced.

These technical changes altered the incidence of locomotor disorders. The new wing paddle, which

gets "stuck" in the water, introduces a much higher strain of the muscles of the arms, and primarily the muscles around the shoulder region. In the adaptation period, the number of muscle, tendon, and joint injuries increased by leaps and bounds. Later, following the adaptation of the muscular system, the number of injuries returned to the previous level. Due to narrower boats, injuries of trunk muscles are more frequent, as these muscles tend to be overloaded in attempts to maintain balance and stability.

Hungarian national team data

The author analyzed the injuries in Olympic flat-water boats at 200, 500, and 1000 m distances as well as marathon distances (35–38 km). The Olympic flatwater team had approximately 35–40 members, and the junior team 45–50 members. The marathon national teams were about half as large. These numbers were subject to change, but the total number was 120–140 persons yearly on average. Therefore, injuries and damage of about 130 competitors were analyzed yearly. The analysis included the 20-year period of 1981–2001. The average training time is 4.5 hours daily, 5–6 times a week (depending on the age of the competitor, the discipline, and the preparation cycle). Competitors train 45 weeks each year, accumulating approximately 1000 hours of activity. In the 20-year period, we analyzed a training program of more than 2.5 million hours. An injury was defined as an

Table 8.1 Changes in Olympic champions' performances between 1964–1984 and 1984–2004.

	1964 result in seconds	1984 result in seconds	Improvement compared to 1964 results (%)	2004 result in seconds	Improvement compared to 1984 results (%)
W K1 500 m	133	118	11.3	108	8.5
W 200 m freestyle swimming	131[a]	119	9.2	118	0.8
M K1 1000 m	237	225	5.1	205	8.9
M K4 1000 m	194	182	6.2	177	2.8
M 1500 m running	218	212	2.8	214	−0.94
M C1 1000 m	275	246	10.6	226	8.1
W 400 m freestyle swimminng	252	231	8.3	223	3.5

[a] 1968 data; no competition in 1964.
1, Single; 4, four-person; C, canoe; K, kayak; M, men; W, women.

occurrence at training or competition, causing at least one day of absence from ordinary training. There were 7914 cases.

Injury rates

This retrospective study of injuries showed that the injury rate by hours of exposure was 3.17 injuries per 1000 hours. Kayaking and canoeing have low incidence rates of injuries. Most of these are minor, and many of them are preventable. All things considered, kayaking and canoeing are safe sports. Most injuries (7423, or 93.8%) occurred during training. The injuries were equally distributed between women and men. Overuse injuries predominated in the preseason period and at the end of the competitive season.

Canoeing is a cyclical, noncontact sport. Therefore, acute or traumatic injuries are relatively rare; the majority of them happen during dryland training, such as weightlifting, running, cross-country skiing, cycling, and so on. Overuse injuries are very common because of the eccentric, cyclical loading repeated in the same joint position several thousand times during every training session. This high-level loading over a long period results in a series of microtraumas and the accumulation of these results in the overuse injuries. In comparison to the literature, the probability of injuries in canoeing is relatively low. Compared to other sports, this is very favorable (Table 8.2).

Incidence of injuries

Injuries were classified in three categories: minor – causing an absence from training of less than 3 days; moderate – causing an absence between 4 and 10 days; and major – causing an absence of 11 or more days.

The overwhelming majority of injuries are minor ones (Table 8.3). Severe injuries happen during dryland training sessions at a ratio of 8:1. The top athletes are highly motivated, competition is very hard, and being a member of the national team is a financial issue too. Therefore, competitors are not interested in exaggerating their complaints.

There were no significant differences when comparing the incidence of injuries between women and men. Similarly, there were no differences between competitors in Olympic distances and those in the marathon. Olympic years are exceptional, as competitors, motivated by starting in the Olympic Games, suffer more overuse injuries. In contradiction to all this, there were differences between kayakers and canoeists as well as between adults and junior competitors. As women have been canoeing for a relatively short time, no conclusions can be drawn regarding the incidence of their injuries (Table 8.4).

The higher vulnerability of canoeists can be explained by their movements and asymmetry; the cause of the higher vulnerability of juniors can be lack of self-control and the fact that their coaches are less experienced.

Table 8.3 Incidence of injuries suffered during kayaking and canoeing and during dryland training.

	%	Kayaking and canoeing	Dryland training
Minor (1–3 days)	82	1	1
Moderate (4–10 days)	11	1	3
Major (≥11 days)	7	1	8

Table 8.2 Incidence of injuries in different sports (no. per 1000 hours).

Soccer (women)	Engström	15.5
Soccer (men)	Junge	8.5
Ice hockey	Lorentzon	39.9
Orienteering	Johansson	3.0
Kayaking and canoeing	Present source	3.2

Table 8.4 Ratios of injuries.

Groups in comparison	Ratios of injuries
Kayaking: women vs. men	1:0.98
Flatwater vs. marathon	1:0.96
Men's canoeing vs. men's kayaking	1:1.22
Adult competitors vs. junior competitors	1:1.27

Common orthopedic injuries

Trunk: muscles

As with other parts of the body, sprains and partial tears can occur in trunk muscles. They can happen during both paddling and supplementary training. According to my experiences, the mm. longissimus dorsi, trapezius, and latissimus dorsi are affected primarily. These injuries occur during supplementary (weightlifting) training and under adverse weather conditions (gusts of wind, rough water) above all.

Trunk: spine

In my experience, lumbar spine disorders are very common in canoeists. My coauthors and I reported on this in the *Hungarian Review of Sports Medicine* in 1987. The collective term *canoeists spine syndrome* includes lumbar convex scoliosis at the side of the pulling hand, increase of lumbosacral angle and lumbar lordosis, spondylosis in the dorsolumbar junction, and Baastrup syndrome.

It is very important to recognize spondylolysis, which is a frequent condition in canoeists. In 1986, we examined the incidence of this. *A* stands for the group of national team canoeists in the 1950s and 1960s, and *B* stands for the national team members in 1986. Junior team members in 1986 are marked with *C* (Table 8.5). The average age of beginning paddling became lower, and their careers longer. At the peak of their careers, the members of the B group had been paddling for a period longer than the whole career of A group members. Incidence of spondylolysis in the European population is 4–6%.

Table 8.5 Canoeists' spine disorders: starting date and duration of career.

	A	B	C
Number of cases	14	18	16
Average age at the beginning of paddling (years)	15	12.1	11.9
Average period of paddling (years)	14.4	15.9	6.9
Scoliosis (no.)	8	13	12
Average angle of the scoliosis	4	8	7
Spondylolysis (no.)	2	9	5

In canoeists, it is several times higher: in group B, it was 50%, and in the junior group C, it was >30%.

A slipped disc occurred in two kayakers (one girl and one boy) during the 20 years of the study. The girl, after discectomy, recovered to win a gold medal in double kayak at the Marathon World Championship.

Upper limb: shoulder

Rotator cuff injury and impingement syndrome are common in overuse injuries in canoeing. These shoulder injuries are often managed conservatively, but if surgery is indicated, the goal is the enlargement of the subacromial space. This is accomplished by partial removal of the acromion and subacromial burse. If the rotator cuff is torn, this requires surgical repair (Figure 8.1).

Shoulder subluxation and dislocation occur more often in slalom, although they are not excluded in sprint either. The usual treatment in shoulder dislocation is surgical reconstruction of injured labrum and other structures after reposition, followed by gradual rehabilitation (Figures 8.2 and 8.3).

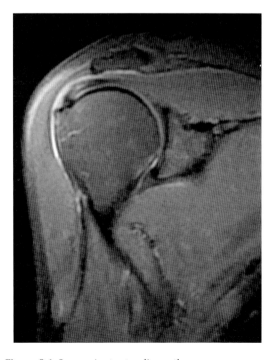

Figure 8.1 Supraspinatus tendinopathy.

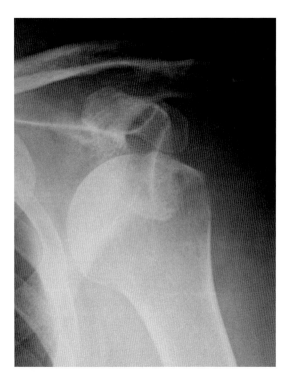

Figure 8.2 Anterior shoulder dislocation.

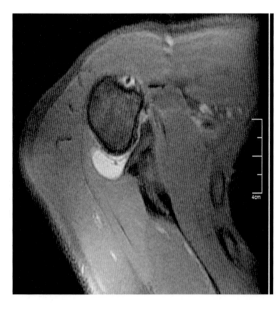

Figure 8.3 Glenoid labral tear.

Tears of the m. pectoralis major are also well-known; these occur with strength training. In this case, the torn tendon needs surgical reconstruction; a long period of rehabilitation is necessary, but return to competitive canoeing is possible (Figure 8.4).

Upper limb: forearm, wrist, and hand

One of the major chronic problems is tendinitis of the wrist extensors. The biomechanical analysis explained that paddling needs power of the pulling hand. Gripping in kayaking and steering in canoeing need forearm work, too. This can cause many forearm and wrist complaints. Paddling in itself and aggressive gripping and steering cause local tenderness, crepitus, and swelling over the overused tendons. Power, generated by body rotation and shoulder muscles, is transferred to the blade by the forearm. In some countries, these complaints are frequent in the period between February and April, when the environmental conditions allow return to paddling after a long non-paddling period. This problem develops in junior olympic-distance team members most often, not in marathon-distance paddlers. In younger competitors, the adaptation of forearm muscles and tendons is slower, paddling technique is worse, and coaches have less experience. Training in indoor paddling tanks or with mechanical or rubber rope simulators is suitable for general training, but not suitable for practicing balance keeping and proper technique.

De Quervain tenosynovitis and carpal tunnel syndrome have been reported in this population. After the winter period, at the beginning of paddling season, a frequent injury is inflammation of the tendons of the flexing muscles of the hands and the ganglion evolving at the metacarpophalangeal and interphalangeal joints. After a long break without paddling, blisters can develop, and prevention of infection is important. The callus (horny skin caused by the shaft of the paddle) at the bottom of the thumb is another characteristic phenomenon, although it does not affect paddling (Figure 8.5).

(a)

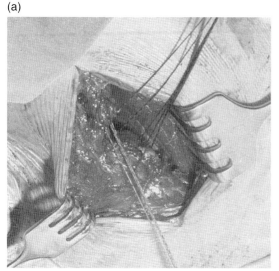

(b)

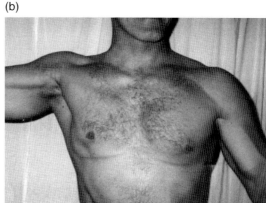

Figure 8.4 (a,b) Rupture of the m. pectoralis major.

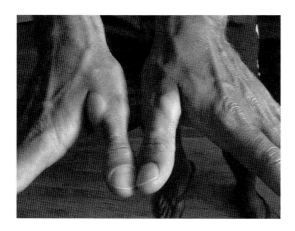

Figure 8.5 Callus on the hands.

Lower limb: pelvis

Ischial bursitis is difficult to distinguish from insertional tendinitis of the hamstring muscles. The pain is localized at the ischial tuberosity and caused by pressure from the hard kayak seat. Treament is conservative, and occasionally an injection of corticosteroid is necessary.

Femoro acetabular impingement (FAI) has become common among canoeists lately. FAI generally occurs in three forms: pincer, cam, and mixed. The *pincer form* describes a situation where the acetabulum has too much coverage surface of the femoral head. The overcoverage generally exists along the front-top part of the acetabulum and results in the labral cartilage being "pinched" between the anterior femoral head–neck junction and the rim of the acetabulum. The pincer form is most often secondary to retroversion, a turning back of the acetabulum; profunda, a socket that is too deep; or protrusio, a situation where the ball extends into the pelvis. The *cam form* shows that the relationship between the femoral head and neck is not perfectly round (i.e. it is aspherical). Loss of roundness results in abnormal contact between the head and acetabulum. The cam and pincer forms may exist together, and this is called *mixed impingement*.

Cartilage damage, early hip arthritis, labral tears, hyperlaxity of the hip joint, subspinous impingement, sports hernias, ischiofemoral impingement, and low back pain: all of these diagnoses can be accompanied by FAI, and FAI can hide in their background (Figure 8.6).

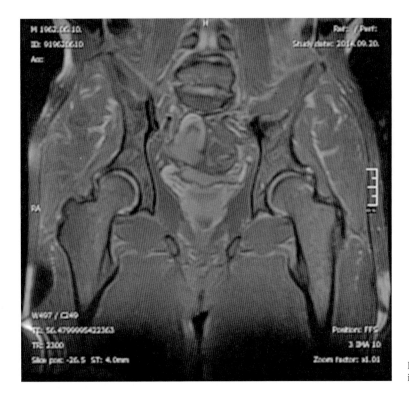

Figure 8.6 Femoroacetabular impingement.

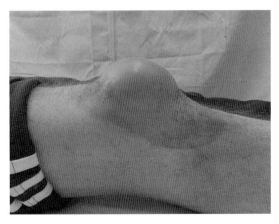

Figure 8.7 Prepatellar bursitis.

Lower limb: knee

Prepatellar bursitis occasionally happens in canoeists in the "down" knee. This needs to be drained (and, rarely, excised) if the problem is recurrent. Patellofemoral pain and chondromalacia also occur in the canoeist (Figure 8.7).

Lower limb: ankle and foot

These parts of the body are infrequently loaded in kayaking and canoeing, so injuries happen only during supplementary training, except for the callus on kayakers' heels (similar to the disorder at the bottom of the thumb).

Prevention and therapy

In kayaking and canoeing, the most common muscle and joint injuries are preventable. Prevention and treatment of the injuries, including overuse injuries, of kayakers and canoeists are not different from prevention and treatment of similar injuries of athletes in other sports.

Since stretching has been used routinely, the incidence of minor muscle injuries has decreased by 25%, and the incidence of moderate muscle injuries has decreased by 10%.

It is very important to emphasize that aptitude tests are inevitable for prevention, first of all in the case of beginners' spinal columns. Paying attention to small (or not-so-small) details of technique can prevent many kayak- and canoe-related injuries. Paddling technique includes, for example, the correct kneeling position. It means choosing the proper distance between the foot and the other knee of the canoeists. Teaching and reteaching (in many countries, the climate doesn't permit whole-year paddling) is the coach's job. Choosing length of the paddle and width of the blade, first of all for beginners and changing these parameters later when the competitor's muscle strength increases, is the coach's job.

Massage before and after training, pre-workout stretching of specific muscles, and warmups both on land and on the water are very important. Unfortunately, even top-level competitors are inclined to neglect this.

Weightlifting, which is a crucial part of training programs throughout the year, is responsible for many injuries. At weightlifting training, the optimal weight, the number of repetitions, and resting time should be chosen correctly. This is a responsibility of the coach. But athletes often do overwork, which can cause first of all muscle injuries. Treatment includes rest and modified training methods (e.g. swimming and/or biking for aerobic training), nonsteroid anti-inflammatory drugs, muscle relaxants, physiotherapy (ultrasound, heat, iontophoresis, magnetic fields, and shock-wave therapy), ice for acute injuries, immobilizing for serious forearm tendinitis, and so on. A discussion with the coach about paddling technique, choosing equipment, and related topics is often warranted.

For example, when the paddle is too long, the power generated by muscles is transferred on a very long lever that can cause many overuse injuries, such as tendinopathies, insertiopathies, tenosynovitis of forearm, and so on. Good equipment and proper paddling technique are very important.

Preparticipation screening and aptitude tests for beginners, adolescents, and master athletes are important medical responsibilities.

Bibliography

Chong-hoon, L. and Ki-jeong, N. (2012). Analysis of the kayak forward stroke according to skill level and knee flexion angle. *Int J BioSci BioTech* 4 (4): 41–48.

Dobos, J., Csépai, D., and Moldvai, I. (2005). Acute and overuse injuries in elite kayakers and canoeists. *Hung Rev Sports Med* 46: 199–211.

Dobos, J., Massányi, L., Somogyvári, K., and Csépai, D. (1987). Analysis of low back deformations of elite canoeists. *Hung Rev Sports Med* 28 (3–4): 227–232.

Dobos, J. and Pavlik, A. (2011). Locomotor anamnesis of the Hungarian Olympic team of Beijing. *Hung Rev Sports Med* 22 (4): 129–144.

Du Toit, P., Sole, G., Bowerbank, P., and Noakes, T.D. (1999). Incidence and causes of tenosynovitis of the wrist extensors in long distance paddle canoeists. *Br J Sports Med* 33: 105–109.

Fiore, D.C. and Houston, J.D. (2001). Injuries in whitewater kayaking. *Br J Sports Med* 35: 235–241.

Kameyama, O., Shibano, K., Kawakita, H. et al. (1999). Medical check of competitive canoeists. *J Orthop Sci (Japan)* 4 (4): 243–249.

Kizer, K. (1987). Medical aspects of white-water kayaking. *Phys Sportsmed* 15: 128–137.

Walsh, M. (1985). Preventing injury in competitive canoeists. *Phys Sportsmed* 13 (9): 120–129.

Chapter 9
Paracanoe

John Edwards[1], Anna Bjerkefors[2], Johanna Rosen[2], and Olga Tarassova[2]

[1]ICF Paracanoe Committee, Mississippi Hills, ON, Canada

[2]Swedish School of Sport and Health Sciences (GIH), Laboratory of Biomechanics and Motor Control, Stockholm, Sweden

Introduction and history

Paddlers with impairments are not a new experience for the sport of canoeing. These paddlers have long known that canoeing, and specifically kayaking, is well suited to those with lower limb impairments. This is due to the obvious fact it is a seated sport. Historic photographs from mid-twentieth-century France attest to this fact (Figures 9.1 and 9.2). For many years, many paddling clubs throughout the world have had individual members who made their own adaptations to pursue paddling for a recreational purpose. Very few activities led to competitions.

Notably, the British Canoe Union (now British Canoeing) for many years included persons with impairments in local and national competitions in kayaking. They followed and still follow a *time-band method*. This is described as permitting paddlers to perform within time-bands. This has the advantage of permitting all impairment classes to compete together, with the only distinction being performance on the water. This is a very inclusive approach. The disadvantage is the potential for manipulation of performances to remain in certain time-bands regardless of true ability.

Likewise, the French Federation of CanoeKayak was active in the promotion of "Handi-Kayak" recreational kayaking in many of its clubs as part of a social agenda to promote sport as a vehicle for social inclusion in French society through sport. In the first decade of the twenty-first century, the Italian and Canadian CanoeKayak Federations were also exploring increasing the participation of persons with impairments in their clubs and competitions.

Paracanoeing has been a recent project of the International Canoe Federation (ICF). In 2004–2008, the ICF distributed questionnaires to member federations in order to measure interest. In March 2008, CanoeKayak Canada organized an international conference, in Montreal, for Paddlers with a Disability. It was sanctioned by the ICF, and Brazil, France, Hungary, Italy, the USA, and Canada sent official delegates. Unofficial delegations were sent from Great Britain and New Zealand. Representatives from the International Va'a Federation's (IVF) adaptive paddling program also attended. This organization had included events for adaptive paddling in their biannual World Championships since 2004.

The conference concluded with a final report, which emphasized the following Principles and Goals:

Principles

- *ICF PaddleALL/PaddleAbility program will address both intellectual and physical disabilities*
  - While the catalyst for the conference has been the Paralympic Games, the PaddleALL movement

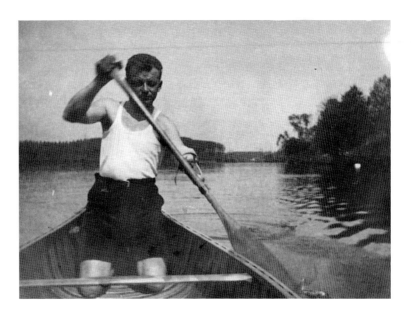

Figure 9.1 Early photo of a single canoe (C1) paddler with a left upper-extremity prosthesis.

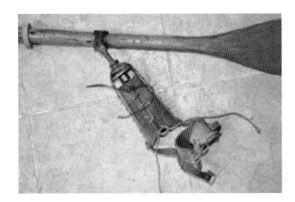

Figure 9.2 Upper-extremity canoe prosthesis with attachment to paddle.

needs to address the needs of all persons with a disability, whether physical or intellectual.

• *Functional and positive approach aligned with World Health Organization protocols and International Paralympic Committee (IPC) classification code*
  • The entire program needs to reflect WHO standards for sports and activities for persons with a disability.
• *Gender-balanced program*
  • As this is a new initiative and program for the ICF, it needs to be gender balanced at the onset.

• *Build a strong foundation for PaddleALL sport development at base of pyramid*
  • For the program to be sustainable in the long term, it needs to have a strong foundation at canoe/kayak clubs, in regions and in nations with resourceful use of existing equipment, quality coaching leadership, awareness promotion, and so on.
• *Work with existing Games and Organizations*
  • Partnerships should be developed with existing Games and the many organizations that promote sport for persons with a disability.
• *Use existing canoe/kayak equipment to promote opportunities for people with disabilities*
  • Rapid expansion of national programs will be facilitated by using existing stable boats that canoe/kayak clubs currently possess or are readily attainable and that can also be used by other types of paddlers (e.g. novices, masters, etc.).
  • Canoe/kayak encompasses many boat types, which will enable this principle.
• *International sharing of technology of coaching, and resources; knowledge transfer*
  • To build the program quickly, all nations must share their experiences and resources. There needs to be an open sharing of information.

- *PaddleALL shall be inclusive*
  - All paddlesports need to be involved in PaddleALL – flatwater canoe and kayak, slalom, dragon boat, outrigger, and so on – because each boat type presents technical opportunities. A unified and coordinated worldwide approach will be the most broadly successful.

Goals (for the International Paralympic Committee)

- *Inclusion of canoe/kayak events in the 2012 Paralympic Games*
  - This goal was an overarching goal at that time. There were indications the IPC would consider a sport such as canoe/kayak as an exhibition sport for the 2012 Summer Paralympic Games if a credible application meeting minimum standards were coordinated in sufficient time. Given the tremendous advantages that inclusion in the 2012 Paralympic Games would have provided, the conference supported this goal as paramount.
- *Both canoe and kayak*
  - Since ICF is the governing body for canoe and kayak, the conference endorsed the goal that events for both canoe and kayak should be included.
- *Gender balanced*
  - PaddleALL is an initiative to, in effect, begin an entirely new ICF program. Since there is clear international direction to all sports from the International Olympic Committee (IOC) to provide gender balance within sports, PaddleALL should be gender balanced from the beginning.
- *Meaningful international competition (rigorous)*
  - Competitions should be "competitive" and serious as opposed to being "participatory"; in other words, identical to the standards of current ICF competition: boat classification standards, rigorous rules, officiating protocols, award protocols, and so on. It should be treated as seriously as mainstream ICF competitions. Competitions should also be integrated into existing mainstream competitions.
- *ICF needs to meet IPC Standards for Inclusion*
  - 18 countries and 3 continents
- *Wide variety of disability groups*

- Sports that offer competitive opportunities for a wide variety of disability groups are more attractive to the IPC than sports that offer opportunities to fewer groups. Currently, of the 27 IPC sports, only field athletics and swimming offer opportunities for all disability groups. At this time, it is not known how many disability groups can be served by rowing, which is formally on the program of the IPC for the first time in London 2012 as a full medal sport. Canoe kayak has the ability to address all major disability groups, particularly through the use of team boats. In this regard, team boats are very attractive.
- *Unified worldwide approach*
  - The approach to the IPC needs to be focused, strong, and worldwide. As the lead worldwide paddlesport organization, ICF should be the lead organization. Equally, from the conference proceedings, it is apparent that outrigger paddling, particularly in the USA and Italy, has demonstrated impressive programs.

    From the technical perspective, the outrigger canoe presents the characteristics of a boat, which could be successful. The conference recognized the political perspective about the outrigger (Va'a) canoe since there is a separate international organization (IVF), which is specifically organized to coordinate international competitions for it. The political aspects of recommending the outrigger for PaddleALL in the Paralympic Games were felt to be beyond the scope of the conference. However, the presentations at the conference clearly indicate the potential that a dialogue between the ICF and the IVF might bear significant promise in three areas: (i) It would provide a stable canoe option, (ii) its team configurations can address multiple disabled groups, and (iii) it would draw Australasia and Pacific Rim countries into an ICF-led program, thus strengthening the ICF bid.

At the 2008 ICF Congress in November, the report from the conference was accepted. The ICF Canoeing For All Committee, under the new chairmanship of John Edwards (of Canada), was given the responsibility to initiate "adaptive paddling" with the initial goal of events at the

2009 Canoe Sprint World Championships in Dartmouth, Canada. The Canoeing For All Committee focused its efforts on expanding participation in specific defined events in order to align with the general directions of the IPC. This goal was achievable and highly beneficial as it made funding available from National Paralympic Committees for paracanoeing. In the period from 2009 until 2014, the paracanoe program made numerous changes and initiatives to achieve IPC recognition. The IPC also changed its minimum number of participating countries to 24 for the 2016 Games. Before international competition could be held, key decisions were made by the ICF:

- Agreement between ICF and IVF reached
  - ICF would remain in the lead, with IVF supporting the initiatives. IVF would have authority over the Va'a boat standards.
- 200 m race distance defined
  - At the same time, the 200 m race distance was adopted for canoe sprint as an Olympic distance. The distance has naturally led to close and exciting races.
- Decision to not include a visually impaired category or intellectual disability category
  - This decision was made for international competitions only. It was driven by a need to provide a focus for ICF in order to strengthen an application for IPC recognition. Once initial inclusion was achieved and events solidified, expansion into other impairments would be explored. National Federations have the authority to encourage wider participation at the national Level. For example, CanoeKayak Canada has developed rules for visually impaired paddlers.
- Kayak boat standard with a minimum width requirement was established
  - ICF adopted a kayak boat standard, which is identical to the ICF canoe sprint kayak standard with one important difference. The width was established at 50 cm and measured 10 cm from the bottom of the hull. This width standard was adopted to provide better stability for the boat when compared to the Olympic canoe sprint kayak. It was based upon an informal kayak touring boat common to parts of Europe. It was also based upon the need to make the sport highly accessible to all potential paracanoe athletes at

all ages and the realization that these boat models already existed at the club level as novice introductory kayaks. This decision has been critical for the rapid growth of paracanoeing.

- Va'a boat standard defined
  - The IVF submitted definitions of rules to the ICF for adoption and promulgation.
- Adaptive equipment
  - Adaptive equipment is not regulated by the ICF. ICF is committed to the principle of letting athletes use whatever equipment deemed necessary to paddle effectively. Equally, the reverse is also true: no athlete would be further disabled through the regulation of adaptive equipment.
- Events
  - Originally, the ICF included tandem and single events. The tandem-event crews, which required mixed gender and mixed abilities, were very difficult to organize due to athletes being older with established lives and thus being unable to relocate to do the necessary training together. This was the case at the international level and would be even more difficult at the national level. Since a strong and robust competitive system needs to have common events from the domestic to the international level, the decision was taken to focus upon single events only. This added events to the program. However, participation has grown strongly since athletes find training on an individual basis easier to accommodate.
- Classification system accepted.
  - The IPC accepted a new sport-specific classification system for kayaking at their board meeting in January 2015. They did not accept the proposed classification system for Va'a. The development of evidence-based sport-specific classification systems is a core goal of the IPC. New sports are expected to comply from their first acceptance into the Paralympic movement. Both paratriathlon and paracanoe had to achieve this goal prior to the Rio 2016 Paralympic Games. Existing Paralympic sports are working toward this goal.

The ICF made a significant investment in time and money to achieve the new system. It is further committed to continue research to develop an acceptable Va'a classification system in time to support the inclusion of Va'a events in the 2020 Tokyo Paralympic Games.

Worldwide growth of paracanoeing

At the 2009 Canoe Sprint World Championships, 27 paracanoeists from seven federations participated. Early participating federations were Brazil, Canada, France, Great Britain, Portugal, Italy, and the USA. However, many federations were watching the initiation of paracanoe events with great interest. At the 2010 Canoe Sprint World Championships, 67 paracanoeists from 28 federations participated. The ICF applied to the IPC for inclusion in the Rio 2016 Paralympic program. This was awarded to the ICF in November 2010. Two conditions were noted: ICF would continue to grow worldwide participation, and a sport specific classification system would be developed and implemented (Figure 9.3).

At the conclusion of 2014, 36 federations attended the 2014 World Championships in Moscow, 11 federations had attended the World Championships between 2010 and 2013, five more federations had attended continental championships, and eight more federations had invested in coaching courses, invested in classification courses, and/or received paracanoe boats for international competition. From a continental perspective, all continents were involved with multiple federations. See Figures 9.4 and 9.5.

The rapid growth of paracanoeing in only a very short time is truly remarkable. This growth has also meant the ICF met the even higher standards (32 countries) to be included as a sport on the 2020 Tokyo Paralympic program. Specific events were determined in 2017. The effort has been a significant display of teamwork among all the ICF Continental Associations and ICF member federations.

This success has led to further discussions with the recreational, tourism, and medical sectors on

Participation numbers
63 WORLD-WIDE FEDERATIONS

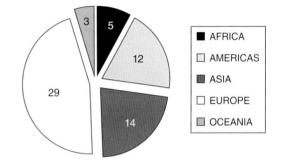

- ■ AFRICA
- □ AMERICAS
- ■ ASIA
- □ EUROPE
- ▨ OCEANIA

Figure 9.4

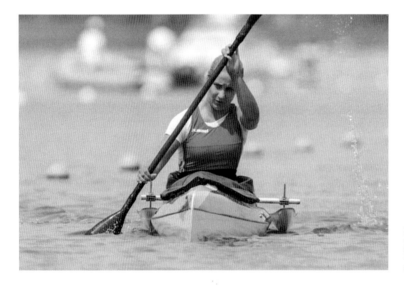

Figure 9.3 Female single kayak (K1) paddler. Note modification to the kayak to provide additional stability.

Participation numbers

63 FEDERATIONS IN PARACANOE

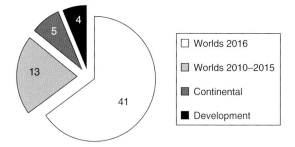

- ☐ Worlds 2016
- ☐ Worlds 2010–2015
- ■ Continental
- ■ Development

Figure 9.5

the benefits of paracanoeing and the larger possibilities of canoeing for all persons with impairments. The future is bright for persons with impairments who wish to explore the world of paddling, both recreational and competitive. The ICF has opened up a world of possibilities through its determined advocacy of paracanoeing (Figure 9.6).

EVIDENCE-BASED CLASSIFICATION FOR PARAKAYAK

Anna Bjerkefors, Johanna Rosén, and Olga Tarassova
Swedish School of Sport and Health Sciences (GIH), Laboratory of Biomechanics and Motor Control, Stockholm, Sweden

The paracanoe classification system that was used between 2009 and 2014 included three classes: Arms (A), Trunk and Arms (TA), and Legs, Trunk, and Arms (LTA). The A class included athletes with the highest impairments, who typically only had function in their arms, or did not have an elbow and wrist joints. The TA class typically had function in their arms and trunk but not in the legs, or did not have a wrist joint. The LTA class were athletes with the least impairment and typically had function in their arms and trunk and partial function in their legs, or loss of at least three fingers. This system was adapted from the pararowing classification system and did not have any research supporting the definitions of the classes. The system was based on

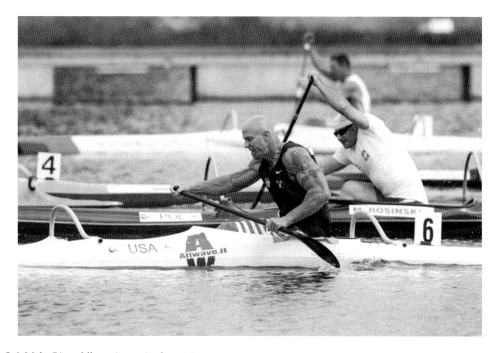

Figure 9.6 Male C1 paddler using a single outrigger canoe.

physical tests assessing muscle strength and joint range of motion (ROM) for upper limbs and lower limbs, where the function was scored from 0 to 5. Three trunk tasks were used to assess the trunk function and were scored from 0 to 2. The system also consisted of technical observations during paddling on an ergometer and on water. The minimal eligibility criteria to be able to compete in paracanoe were to have either (i) at least full loss of three fingers on one hand, (ii) at least partial foot amputation, or (iii) a permanent loss of at least 10 points on one limb or 15 points across two limbs in the physical assessment tests.

In recent years, the IPC has highlighted the importance of an evidence-based classification system for all athletes with physical impairments, to control the impact of impairment on the outcome of competition. The ICF has therefore supported a research project to evaluate, develop, and present a report to the IPC representing a validated and evidence-based classification system for paracanoers. The overall purpose of new classification systems is to achieve the purpose of promoting participation in sport by people with disability. The purpose of the research is to identify how much impairment of varying type, location, and severity impact the kayak paddling performance by:

Defining eligibility: to be eligible to compete in paracanoe, athletes must have an impairment that:

- is one of the three eligible types of impairment (impaired muscle power, impaired range of motion, or limb deficiency),
- is permanent in nature (i.e. will not resolve in the foreseeable future regardless of physical training, rehabilitation, or other therapeutic interventions), and
- causes a sufficient level of activity limitation: the athlete must have an impairment defined by the minimum eligibility criteria.

Minimizing the impact of impairment on the outcome of competition:

- The athletes should succeed because they have the most favorable combination of anthropometric, physiological, and psychological attributes.
- Athletes who succeed will do so because they are stronger in these areas, rather than because they have an impairment that causes less activity limitation.

To create an evidence-based classification system for parakayak, research was conducted by our research group. The results helped in creating/modifying the assessment tests, determining the number of classes, how the classes were defined, and defining the minimal eligibility criteria used in classification for parakayak.

The assessment tests used for classification of parakayak athletes

The first step in creating the new Paralympic classification system for parakayak was to define the joint ROMs in elite able-bodied athletes when paddling on a kayak ergometer. It was important to define these values to ensure that the physical assessment tests used for classification of parakayak athletes actually assess the relevant ROM required for the sport. Since the paddling movement is complex with three-dimensional (3D) upper-body movements during water and aerial phase time, a 3D kinematic analysis during the kayak paddling was chosen as a method to analyze the sport-specific ROM. This analysis was also conducted on elite parakayak athletes to investigate the relation between power output and joint angles.

Ten elite international-level able-bodied kayakers and 41 elite national- or international-level parakayakers with impairments affecting the trunk and/or legs were tested. 3D kinematic data and 3D power output were collected while the athletes were paddling on a kayak ergometer at low, high, and maximal intensity levels.

Maximal and minimal peak joint angle for flexion and extension and total ROM were calculated for the shoulder, elbow, wrist, trunk, hip, knee, and ankle joints. Additionally, maximal and minimal peak joint angle and the ROM were calculated for shoulder abduction and rotation, for trunk rotation and lateral bending, and for ulnar and radial deviation.

Correlations were calculated between all joint angles and power output for males and females. From these results, it was evident that sitting in a forward flexed trunk position, being able to rotate the trunk and pelvis, and moving the hip, knee, and ankle joints in a pumping movement pattern are important for producing power output. Thus, evaluating trunk and leg function is crucial in parakayak athletes with full upper-limb function.

Trunk and leg tests

The second step in creating the new Paralympic classification system was to develop a trunk test and to modify the leg test. Currently, there are no established clinical methods for examining motor function in the trunk muscles in individuals with impaired muscle power, for example following a spinal cord injury (SCI). However, it has been incorporated into classification of trunk function for Paralympic athletes such as in wheelchair rugby and Nordic skiing. Recent research has examined the accuracy of using manual examination to determine abdominal muscle function in persons with impaired muscle power (i.e. individuals with SCI). Therefore, a trunk test to determine the trunk function in para-athletes was developed and implemented. The trunk test includes a manual muscle test (MMT) and a functional trunk test (FTT). The MMT consists of seven different trunk muscle tasks: trunk flexion, trunk lumbar extension, trunk and hip extension, trunk rotation to the left and right, and trunk bending to the left and right. Athletes' abdominal muscles are individually scored on a scale from 0 to 2. The load of the exercise can be adjusted by changing the position of the arms (Figure 9.7).

After the MMT is performed, the athletes are asked to complete the FTT while sitting unsupported. The test includes (i) static tasks: sitting upright with arms across chest and with arms outstretched in four directions; (ii) dynamic tasks: moving trunk through a range of motion in six directions; (iii) perturbation tasks: push and recovery from six directions; and (iv) perturbation tasks while the athlete is sitting on a wobble cushion: push and recovery from six directions. The tasks are graded from 0 to 2: clearly fails (0), in doubt (1), and succeeds (2). The scores for all tests are summed to a total sum score, which can range from 0 to 84 points.

The previous leg test used for classification of leg function consisted of seven different bilateral tasks scored on a 0–5 scale: hip, knee, and ankle flexion/ extension strength and ROM, as well as a standing squat test. The new leg test consists of seven bilateral tests evaluating hip, knee, and ankle muscle strength through the sport-specific ROM obtained from the 3D kinematic analysis on able-bodied athletes. The tests are graded on a 0–2-point scale with a maximal total score of 28 points. The previous standing squat test was replaced by a sitting single leg press test.

On-water test

The technical assessment during paddling was previously only an observation on water and on an ergometer, which included 13 items that were not scored. The new technical assessment is now a scored on-water test that consists of six items that are scored

(a)

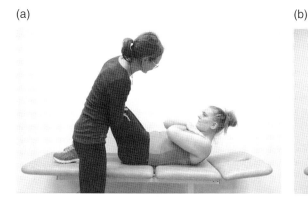

(b)

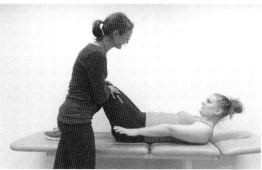

Figure 9.7 (a) Trunk flexion in supine with arms crossed over chest (score 2), and (b) arms outstretched in full extension above plane of body (score 1).

from 0 to 2. These six items were chosen based on the results from the 3D kinematic and kinetic analyses of both able-bodied and parakayak athletes. The scored items are left leg movement, right leg movement, balance, trunk posture, trunk rotation, and trunk side flexion. The total score for the on-water test can therefore range between 0 and 12. For a detailed description and a guideline for the Trunk, Leg, and On-water test, please visit the "Paracanoe" section on ICF's webpage (www.canoeicf.com).

The new Paralympic classification system for parakayak

The third step of creating the new Paralympic classification system was to define groups/clusters within the para-athlete group for each assessment test (trunk, leg, and on-water), to further divide the athletes into classes, and to define minimal eligibility. To define the groups/clusters, cluster analyses were performed on the total score for each assessment test. The results showed that there were three clusters for each test. In Figure 9.8, the clusters are further explained.

To further divide the athletes into classes, the cluster scores (1, 2, or 3) from each test are summed into a total classification score, ranging from 3 to 9. Further analyses resulted in there being three different classes. Athletes with the greatest impairment are classified as Kayak Level 1 (KL1) and are typically athletes with no function in either trunk or legs. The second class is called Kayak Level 2 (KL2) and typically includes athletes with limited trunk function and/or limited or no leg function. The third class includes athletes with the least impairments and is called Kayak Level 3 (KL3). The

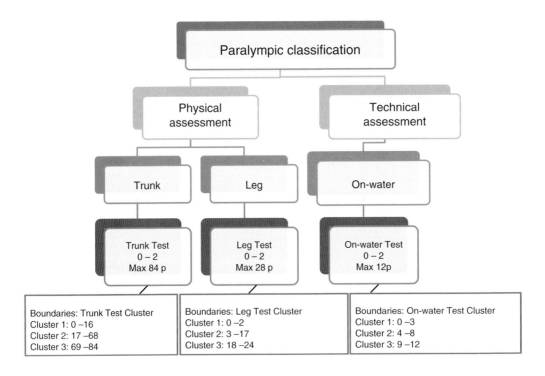

Figure 9.8 For the trunk test, the score ranges for each cluster are 0–16 for cluster 1 (no or limited trunk function), 17–68 for cluster 2 (partial trunk function), and 69–84 for cluster 3 (full or almost-full trunk function). For the leg test, the score ranges for each cluster are 0–2 for cluster 1 (no or limited leg function), 3–17 for cluster 2 (partial leg function), and 18–28 for cluster 3 ("full" leg function; *full leg function* is a term used to define the para-athletes with highest leg function). Please note that the minimal eligibility criterion is set at 24 points, meaning that the athlete needs to have a loss of 4 points. For the on-water test, the score ranges for each cluster are 0–3 for cluster 1, 4–8 for cluster 2, and 9–12 for cluster 3.

athletes in this group typically have near-to-full or full trunk function and limited leg function.

The new minimal eligibility criterion is at least loss of four points in one leg in the physical assessment leg test. This means that, for example, an athlete with no function in one ankle or limited function in one ankle and one knee in the same leg meets the eligibility criterion as a parakayak athlete.

Biomechanical differences between able-bodied and parakayak athletes

To examine differences between the new Paralympic classes and able-bodied athletes, mean angle values of each joint for each class during paddling at high intensity were calculated. The joint ROM of the hip, knee, and foot flexion angles and the trunk and pelvis rotation angles of the able-bodied athletes were significantly different from those of all para-athlete classes. Differences were also seen between the para-athlete classes, where the athletes with greater physical impairment exhibited lower RoMs compared to those with less impairment. This indicates that the new Paralympic classification system for parakayak divides athletes into appropriate groups based on their physical function.

Conclusions

• The range of movement values from the able-bodied group was used as reference values in the sport-specific evidence-based classification system for parakayak athletes.
• During kayaking, sitting in a position of forward trunk flexion and having a greater range of move-

ment in trunk rotation correlate with producing a greater power output.
• Having a greater range of movement in hip, knee, and foot flexion during kayaking correlates with producing a greater power output.
• The new classification system consists of three classes (KL1, KL2, and KL3) into which the athletes are divided, based on the scores from a leg, trunk, and on-water test.

Acknowledgments

We are grateful for all of the help and support we have received from the international paracanoe classifier team, and from athletes and federations, during the process of creating this new evidence-based classification system for parakayak and for the ongoing project for para-Va'a. We would also like to thank the Swedish National Centre for Research in Sports (CIF), the Swedish School of Sport and Health Sciences, and the International Canoe Federation for financial support.

Bibliography

Brown, M.B., Lauder, M., and Dyson, R. (2011). Notational analysis of sprint kayaking: differentiating between ability levels. *Intl J Performance Anal Sport* 11: 171–183.

Limonta, E., Squadrone, R., Rodano, R. et al. (2010). Tridimensional kinematic analysis on a kayaking simulator: key factors to successful performance. *Sport Sci Health* 6: 27–34.

Nilsson, J.E. and Rosdahl, H.G. (2016). Contribution of leg muscle forces to paddle force and kayak speed during maximal effort flat-water paddling. *Intl J Sports Physiol Perform* 11 (1): 22–27.

Tweedy, S.M. and Vanlandewijck, Y.C. (2011). International Paralympic Committee position stand- background and scientific principles of classification in Paralympic sport. *Br J Sports Med* 45: 259–269.

Chapter 10
Exercise performance in masters canoeing athletes

Bo Berglund

Department of Medicine, Karolinska University Hospital, Solna, Sweden

When the modern sports movement developed about 150 years ago, the focus was to improve health and performance in young people. In line with its basic ideas, the Olympic movement still calls "the Youth of the World" to the Olympic Games every four years. However, nowadays the Olympic Charter has changed and promotes sport for all: "the practice of sport is a human right. Every individual must have the possibility of practicing sport in accordance with his or her needs." In parallel with the changes of the Olympic movement, modern countries worldwide promote physical activity for their general populations. The reason is simple: physical activity leads to a win-win situation where the individual improves health and well-being and society reduces healthcare costs. The trend of increased physical activity in the general population is very important, since the number of elderly is increasing worldwide.

In parallel with the number of elderly, the number of middle-aged and older athletes (master athletes) is increasing in many sports. The International Masters Games Association (recognized by the International Canoe Federation [ICF]) is the worldwide representative body for masters sports; it organizes the World Masters Game (since 1985) and encourages all people beyond young adulthood to play sport and to participate in Masters Games with the awareness that

competitive sport can continue throughout life and improve personal fitness.

Recreational canoeing and kayaking are becoming increasingly popular worldwide and can be enjoyed by enthusiasts of all ages. Nowadays, master athletes can compete in racing events such as World Masters Games and other competitions sanctioned by the ICF.

Master athletes strive to maintain and increase performance, and as a consequence training methods and nutritional practices also have improved in this group of athletes. Indeed, the peak exercise performance of master athletes continues to increase, and master athletes have achieved impressive performance. However, declines in athletic performance are inevitable, and the underlying reasons are important to understand. For the purpose of this chapter, the typical athlete is considered old over age 50. By this age, it is usually apparent that an athlete is experiencing several performance-altering physical changes: lower levels of testosterone, lost muscle mass, increased risk of osteopenia and osteoporosis, a greater propensity for weight gain, and lost soft tissue elasticity, with an increased likelihood of injury. The present chapter will focus on the factors responsible for the decline in performance with age and also some medical problems that tend to be accentuated in master athletes.

Canoeing, First Edition. Edited by Don McKenzie and Bo Berglund.
© 2019 International Olympic Committee. Published 2019 by John Wiley & Sons Ltd.

Decline in performance with age

No scientific studies have described the decline in performance with age in master paddlers, so we must rely mainly on information from studies on master athletes involving sports such as swimming, running, and cycling.

In general, peak endurance performance is maintained until about 35 years of age, followed by modest decreases until 50–60 years of age, with progressively steeper reductions thereafter (see also Figure 10.1). The primary reasons why endurance performance declines with age appear to be a combination of aerobic capacity and muscle mass decline. One important factor behind this decline is the reduced production of anabolic hormones. It appears that the loss of functional capacity in master athletes cannot be fully overcome by training, and older athletes may also be limited by the inability to maintain the same volume and intensity of training as young athletes. Also, older athletes appear to respond and recover more slowly to the same training load than do younger athletes. However, it must be realized that some of the changes that come with aging can be the result of a long-standing sedentary lifestyle before a career as a master athlete.

In some sports, the magnitude of decline in endurance performance with age seems to be greater in women than in men. However, such sex differences with age are absent in swimming, where an approximately equal number of men and women train and compete at high levels throughout the age range.

Endurance versus sprinting performance decline

Studies on masters' running world records suggest that performance in distance events declines more rapidly with age than sprinting performance. In line with these observations, master swimmers also seem to have a greater decline in performance in

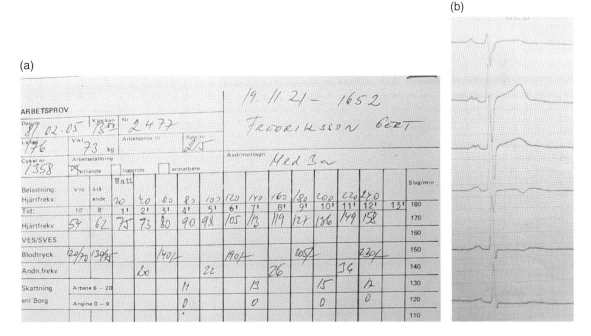

Figure 10.1 (a) Test data from a health evaluation of the late Gert Fredriksson (1919–2006), the world's most successful male Olympic paddler. At age 62, with a body mass index (BMI) = 23.5 and still paddling regularly, he had a $P_{max} = 3.3\,W\,kg^{-1}$ on the cycle ergometer. (b) Electrocardiogram (ECG) was finally diagnosed as athlete's heart.

long-distance events than in short-distance events. Taken together, these observations suggest that endurance performance is indeed more affected by age than sprinting.

However, analysis of track and field records from different age classes showed that for explosive-strength sports such as shotput and discus throwing, declines occur more rapidly with age than in running disciplines, suggesting that "strength deteriorates faster than stamina."

Physiological aspects of decline in endurance exercise performance with age

Based mainly on studies on young endurance athletes, three main physiological determinants of endurance performance have evolved. The first, maximal oxygen uptake (VO_{2max}), is generally considered the major determinant of endurance performance. The second, maximal fractional utilization of VO_{2max}, determines maximal steady-state workload (lactate threshold); and the third factor is exercise efficiency, which relates oxygen demand to workload. The latter physiological parameter, however, is not wholly exclusive from the two others, and their interplay is complex. Some of the underlying physiological mechanisms responsible for the reduction in performance with age in endurance athletes are unclear, particularly so regarding the more specific contribution of central (i.e. cardiac) and peripheral (i.e. oxygen extraction) factors in masters compared with young-adult endurance athletes.

VO_{2max} declines about 10% per decade after age 25–30 years in healthy sedentary adults of both sexes, and the rate of decline with advancing age seems to be similar in master athletes who have continued to train and also were athletes at a young age. The progressive reduction in VO_{2max} appears to be the key physiological mechanism associated with declines in endurance performance with advancing age. In spite of the strong association between VO_{2max} and endurance exercise performance, other factors may contribute. The observation that the rate of decline in endurance performance with age appears to be smaller than the corresponding fall in VO_{2max} is consistent with this idea. It may be that other factors of endurance performance may decline to a lesser extent with advancing age, thus offsetting the effects of the decrease in VO_{2max}.

VO_{2max} is described by Fick's equation:

$$VO_2 = \text{heart rate}(HR) \times \text{stroke volume}(SV) \times K \times (\text{arteriovenous oxygen extraction})$$

It appears that decreases in both maximal central (i.e. cardiac) and peripheral (i.e. oxygen extraction) factors may contribute to a reduced VO_{2max} in older master athletes; see also Table 10.1.

Maximal cardiac output is reduced in older master athletes as compared with young endurance athletes as a result of mainly reductions in maximal HR, and this determinant has been considered the primary mechanism mediating age-related reductions in maximal cardiac output. Maximal HR declines with age, and maximal HR at a given age in master athletes is best described by the equation $HR_{age} = 211 - 0.64 \times age$. However, at least in older

Table 10.1 Oxygen consumption and its determinants at maximal exercise in endurance-trained men.

	Young men (28 years)	Old men (60 years)	Age-related change (%)
Oxygen consumption (ml kg^{-1} min^{-1})	68.2	49.4	28
Cardiac output (l min^{-1})	27	21.7	20
Stroke volume (ml beat^{-1})	147	132	10
Heart rate (beats min^{-1})	184	165	10
A–V difference (ml [100 ml]$^{-1}$)	16.7	15.2	8

Source: Data compiled from four studies; for references, see Tanaka and Seals (2008).

master endurance athletes, there also is a modest reduction of maximal SV by about 10%.

A reduction in peripheral oxygen extraction may also contribute to the decline in VO_{2max}. This factor declines modestly (5–10%) over a span of about 30 years in master endurance athletes.

Lactate threshold is a good predictor of exercise performance in events ranging from about 4 minutes and up. Absolute work rate at lactate threshold declines with age in endurance athletes, but lactate threshold does not appear to change with age when expressed relative to the percentage of VO_{2max}. The latter finding suggests that the contribution of decreases in lactate threshold to reductions in endurance exercise performance with aging may be secondary to decreases in VO_{2max}.

Exercise economy is measured as the steady-state oxygen consumption while exercising at a specific submaximal exercise intensity below the lactate threshold. Among endurance athletes, exercise economy is an important determinant of endurance performance in groups that are more homogeneous than heterogeneous in VO_{2max}. Numerous cross-sectional and longitudinal studies have confirmed that reductions in exercise economy do not contribute significantly to the decreases in endurance exercise performance observed with advancing age.

A number of physiological factors determine exercise economy. One important such factor is the percentage of type I muscle fibers, which is positively related to exercise economy; endurance-trained master athletes seem to have similar muscle fiber distribution as younger endurance athletes. Consistent with this, a two-decade longitudinal study showed that with maintenance of strenuous endurance training, muscle fiber type distribution did not change with age. Therefore, maintenance of muscle fiber type with aging may contribute to the preserved exercise economy of master athletes.

Physiological aspects of decline of sprint exercise performance with age

Sprinting performance at a given age is determined by anaerobic capacity at a young age minus the age-related decline in anaerobic capacity. Short-term muscle power depends on the degradation of adenosine triphosphate (ATP) and its replenishment from phosphocreatine (PCr). The rate of both processes is comparatively high, but as PCr stores are limited and need to be replenished by the slower, oxidative metabolism, the high phosphate-based power can be sustained only for a limited time. Therefore, sprinting performance basically relies upon "anaerobic" mechanisms. Within skeletal muscle, power generation in sprinting performance is mainly by type II muscle fibers, which are specialized in anaerobic power generation, whereas type I fibers mainly are responsible for the aerobic power generation in endurance events. Endurance-trained master athletes may have similar muscle fiber distribution as younger endurance athletes. There are, however, longitudinal studies for ages 65 to 75 years that indicate a decrease of type I content. In light of these considerations, the finding of a more pronounced decline in endurance as compared with sprinting performance with age seems reasonable. Unfortunately, few studies are available on muscle function in master athletes at the fiber level, and no single study has directly compared distance and sprint athletes. To conclude, there are multiple lines of evidence for a fairly linear loss of anaerobic power, equivalent to 1% of the power of a 40-year-old person per year, from the age of 40 onward in athletes as well as in a fit elderly population.

Aspects of training in master athletes

As realized from the information shown in this chapter, master athletes are constantly fighting an uphill battle against the fact of life. Therefore, older athletes must adapt and realize that there is less latitude for mistakes than when they were younger. For example, temporarily cutting back on training will exacerbate problems when the aging athlete once again trains seriously. When younger, the same athlete may well have bounced back quickly from a break in training. So, a critical issue in master athletes is training consistency, and the focus for the aging athlete must be to maintain a broad basic training of different intensities and capacities.

Basically, there are three elements of physical training that can be manipulated to produce fitness, namely workout duration, workout intensity, and workout frequency. In old athletes, there is a tendency to increase duration at the expense of intensity. Workouts become longer and slower as weekly volume becomes the focus of training. The aging athlete needs to do just the opposite if he or she is to perform at a high level despite the aging process. Workouts above 80% intensity factor (just below and above the anaerobic/lactate threshold) with an emphasis on muscular endurance, anaerobic endurance, and sprint power must be included in training programs for two or three sessions a week. This change typically results in shorter training sessions but higher weekly average intensity.

Strength training is one of the best ways that master athletes can build bone density while also stimulating testosterone release to maintain muscle mass. The use of heavy loads with traditional strength training is usually needed, but different types of *body-weight-only* exercises may also be of importance. Strength training should be done frequently and regularly, but it should vary with the season. This type of training will improve the aging athlete's bone and muscle health.

Master athletes, as compared to young athletes, who want to perform at a high level have less latitude for mistakes in the recovery period. With increasing age, adequate sleep is especially important. Sleep regularity, quantity, and quality are necessary to allow the body to cope with training stress, for it is during sleep that the body mainly releases growth hormone and testosterone. Therefore, aging athletes must be very careful not to compromise sleep. If an athlete has to use an alarm clock to wake up in the morning, the sleeping period is too short, and there is a need to go to bed earlier.

After sleep, the second most effective modality for improving recovery is nutrition. There are two primary areas of concern: adequate carbohydrate and protein in the recovery period *immediately* following a long and/or intense workout, and a micronutrient-dense (vitamins and minerals) diet for the remainder of the day. The first requires taking sugar during a long and intense workout (water is all that is needed during short workouts) with starch consumed in the recovery window after exercise. These during-exercise and recovery foods are micronutrient-poor but necessary for rebuilding glycogen stores. Once short-term recovery is achieved, the athlete should reduce the intake of starch and sugar.

Lifestyle aspects of decline in endurance performance with age

Lifestyle factors may contribute to reductions in performance with age in master athletes. Motivation and intrinsic drive to train may be reduced and related to age, and goals underlying the motivation to train may also shift from achieving personal records in younger master athletes to health benefits in older master athletes. In middle age, increases in job- and family-related responsibilities may impinge on the availability of time and energy for intensive training. During this period, longitudinal studies suggest that performance can be fairly well maintained in athletes who continue to train vigorously. An example is given in Figure 10.1. The athlete is Gert Fredriksson, the all-time most successful male Olympic kayaker, who continued to train for many years after his active career.

However, there is no evidence that the necessary high-exercise training load can be maintained for longer periods at older ages. In contrast, available evidence suggests an overall reduction in exercise training load with more advancing age. Therefore, aging-related declines in endurance performance appear to be mediated in large part by a reduction in the intensity and volume of the exercise that can be performed during training sessions.

Medical risks

One factor that contributes to this reduction in exercise training load is the increased prevalence of injury resulting from a high training load at older ages. Typically, the older master athlete will become injured easier, and the injury is likely to heal slower.

Therefore, master athletes must increase their training load slowly over time.

Above the age of 35, coronary heart disease (CHD) is a major medical problem and risk factor for early death in modern society. Elderly recreational paddlers and master athletes encounter more dangers from cold-water environments than young subjects. The reason for this is multifactorial. Firstly, the risk of turn-overs increases with aging due to the fact that balance and mobility also deteriorate with age. Secondly, cardiac arrest, ventricular fibrillation, and other cardiovascular (CV) consequences of hypothermia are accentuated by an underlying CHD. In this context, it must also be noted that arm-work induces higher blood pressure and thus per se increases the risk for CV events, as compared to other sports.

In endurance-type master athletes, the prevalence of atrial fibrillation (an electrical abnormality of the heart associated with irregular rhythm) is increased fivefold in those athletes who have been training for many years (i.e. decades).

Some diseases that can cause transient unconsciousness and inability to maintain balance will increase with age, for example paroxysmal atrial fibrillation (see also the previous paragraph), different types of ventricular arrhythmias, type 2 diabetes, and respiratory problems such as chronic obstructive lung disease. In addition to the diseases per se, many types of medication may also cause this type of problem.

Preparticipation screening is nowadays often performed in elite athletes. However, since the medical risks in master athletes are increased in a multifactorial manner by age, it seems reasonable to include also these elite master athletes in such screening programs.

Bibliography

Ransdell, L.B., Vener, J., and Huberty, J. (2009). Masters athletes: an analysis of running, swimming and cycling performance by age and gender. *J Exerc Sci Fit* 7 (2): S61–S73.

Tanaka, H. and Seals, D.R. (2008). Endurance exercise performance in master athletes: age-associated changes and underlying physiological mechanisms. *J Appl Physiol* 586 (1): 55–63.

Trappe, S.W., Costill, D.L., Vukovich, M.D. et al. (1996). Aging among elite distance runners: a 22-year longitudinal study. *J Appl Physiol* 80 (1): 285–289.

Wright, V.Y. and Perricelli, B.C. (2008). Age-related rates of decline in performance among elite senior athletes. *Am J Sports Med* 36 (3): 443–450.

Chapter 11
Diversity in canoe sport

Don McKenzie[1] and Kari-Jean McKenzie[2]

[1] Division of Sport and Exercise Medicine, The University of British Columbia, Vancouver, BC, Canada

[2] Department of Medicine, The University of British Columbia, Vancouver, BC, Canada

Introduction

No other sport has the diversity of canoeing. As well as the two Olympic disciplines and paracanoe, the sport has many other disciplines that cover a wide range of activities. From long-distance ocean racing on surf skis or Va'a, to acrobatics in standing waves in a river, there is a type of canoeing that is attractive to all who value physical activity and water sports. All competitive disciplines fall under the International Canoe Federation (ICF) governance model and have regular competitions. Technical Committees organize World Cup and World Championship events. Athletes can compete in more than one discipline, and there are strong connections that lead to the Olympic Games. Wildwater, freestyle, marathon, and ocean racing feed the slalom and sprint competitions at the Games.

Canoeing as a form of recreation is one of the fastest growing activities in the world, with at least 53 million recreational paddlers worldwide. Aside from the health benefits of regular physical activity, canoeing is esthetically pleasing, safe, and fun, and it connects you with the environment. It is an attractive activity for all ages. Recently, paddling has been used in the management of patients with chronic disease and forms a unique aspect of healthcare – *canoeing as medicine*.

Women in canoe

The pathway leading to women competing in canoe has been long and tortuous. Although women are highly competitive in kayak and have the same boat skills and technical ability as men in both slalom and sprint, the acceptance of women in Olympic canoe was delayed. Much of this was due to issues related to gender equity in sport but also due to reluctance to accept women as capable of paddling a racing canoe. There was misrepresentation of the risk associated with this discipline. Although it is difficult to comprehend, women were warned that the unilateral movement pattern of Olympic-style canoeing would affect the reproductive organs, causing infertility and injury. This myth has no substance, and women in canoe have been accepted by all National Federations. Injuries that occur in this discipline are the same as with men: shoulder and lumbar spine strain, forearm tendinopathy, and patellofemoral problems in the down knee. Women compete in single canoe (C1) in slalom and C1 and double canoe (C2) in sprint, over distances of 200 m (C1) and 500 m (C2). Women in canoe have achieved medal status in sprint and slalom racing at ICF competitions, and canoeing will be on the program at the 2020 Summer Olympic Games in Tokyo (Figures 11.1 and 11.2; see Tables 1.1 and 1.2).

Canoeing, First Edition. Edited by Don McKenzie and Bo Berglund.

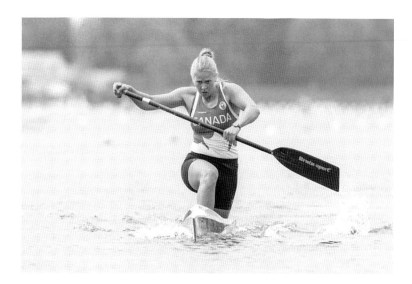

Figure 11.1 Woman single canoe (C1) sprint paddler.

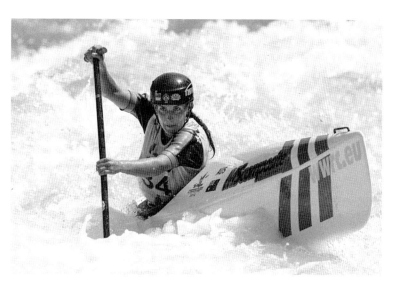

Figure 11.2 Woman C1 slalom paddler.

Marathon

Marathon racing involves long-distance paddling with portages. The start and finish are often in the same location, with the portages set where the public can watch. Women and men compete in marathon races, the distances are varied, and the events are challenged in C1 and single kayak (K1), as well as double kayak (K2) and C2. The classic marathon involves paddling from one location to another, often over different water conditions. Some of

these races are very popular and attract hundreds or even thousands of athletes.

Physiologically, these are primarily aerobic events with some sprinting at the start and finish. The portages involve transporting the boat and paddle over a short distance, getting back in the boat, and continuing to paddle. Wash riding can save valuable energy and is a useful boat skill (Figures 11.3 and 11.4). Substrate availability, hydration, and thermal stress combine with aerobic capacity and race strategy to determine success. Injuries are of the overuse variety; muscle fatigue is

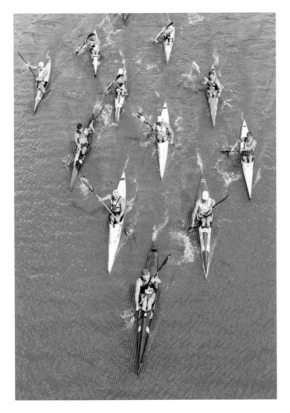

Figure 11.3 Men's single kayak (K1) marathon competition demonstrating wash riding to conserve energy.

the rapid progression of the sport. In 2006, the ICF welcomed canoe freestyle as one of its official disciplines. Athletes have a set time to perform as many different moves and tricks as possible, and they can score additional points for style. Finals are judged over three runs of 45 seconds. The tricks are similar to those seen in freestyle snowboarders, surfers, and skaters, where the athlete completes turns, spins, and flips (Figures 11.5 and 11.6).

Flexibility, strength, and power are necessary prerequisites for performance. Impressive core strength is mandatory to compete. Athletes wear protective gear, as contact with the boat and paddle is possible. Competence in swimming is an essential characteristic. Injuries on the basis of trauma can occur; abrasions and muscle strain are common.

Canoe polo

Canoe polo is played on flat water, often in a swimming pool. Competitions occur indoors or outdoors, and thermal stress can be a concern. The field of play is a $23 \times 35\,m$ rectangle with a goal suspended overhead at each end. The ball used is the same as in water polo, and throwing the ball into the net scores a goal. A team is five players with three additional substitutes. There are two 10-minute halves to a game. At the international level, it combines the speed of sprint with the kayak control of slalom and the ball skills of water polo.

common, and tendinopathy of the forearm, rotator cuff, and shoulder impingement are frequent conditions experienced by these athletes. Stress fractures of the ribs and degenerative changes in the acromioclavicular joint are not uncommon. Master paddlers should be screened for cardiovascular disease.

Canoe freestyle

Freestyle canoeing is growing in popularity. It is contested on a river with standing waves, or stationary features that allow the competitor to perform acrobatic tricks. These are the canoe gymnasts capable of spectacular displays of arrangements and tricks. Boat designs have evolved quickly, improving maneuverability and size and allowing

Players are allowed to push or tip each other into the water, and to ram or ride up on an opponent's boat. There are unique skills, tactics, and equipment. Players wear helmets with a cage to protect the face, and padded vests. The nose and tail of the boat are fitted with impact-absorbing material to prevent injury to the competitors and damage to the boat and paddle. The boat can capsize, and it is necessary to be a competent swimmer. The upper body is used for paddling, and throwing and rotator cuff strain is possible. Generally speaking, in spite of the optics, canoe polo is a low-impact sport, and injury rates are low (Figures 11.7 and 11.8).

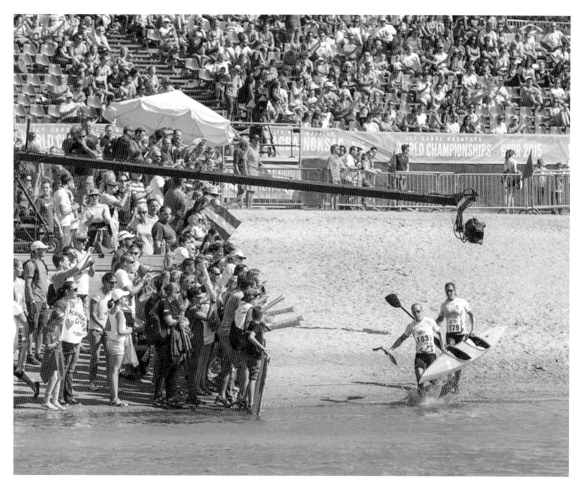

Figure 11.4 Athletes in double kayak (K2) marathon competition during a portage.

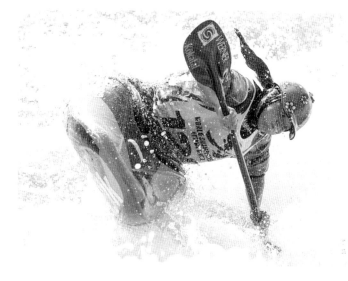

Figure 11.5 Freestyle paddler during competition.

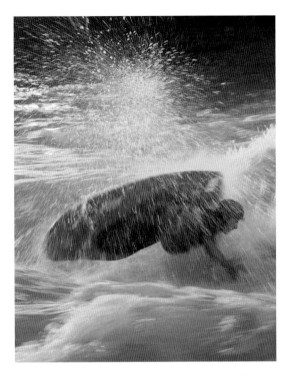

Figure 11.6 Acrobatic moves and tricks in freestyle competition.

Wildwater

Wildwater racing takes place in a demanding, natural environment with fast-moving water, powerful currents, and strong eddies. Competitors must wear protective equipment, as injuries can occur as the athletes race in this challenging environment.

There are two types of competition. In the *classic wildwater* events, athletes race down a course of variable distances with class III to IV whitewater. The performance criterion is time. This is a physically challenging event that requires strength, aerobic capacity, and the ability to "read" the river – to navigate the standing waves, rapids, waterfalls, rocks, and other obstacles.

Sprint wildwater races are conducted on a much shorter course. World Championships have both classic and sprint races for men and women. The categories are K1, C1, and C2 for both genders, in individual and team events (Figures 11.9 and 11.10).

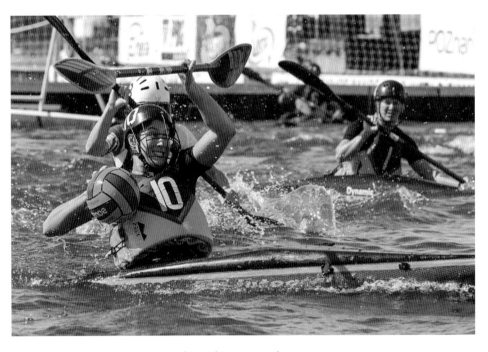

Figure 11.7 Female competitor prepares to try for goal in canoe polo.

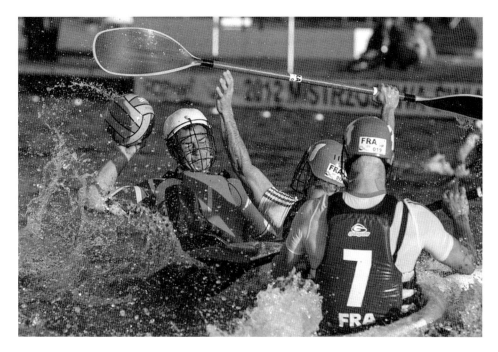

Figure 11.8 Canoe polo competition.

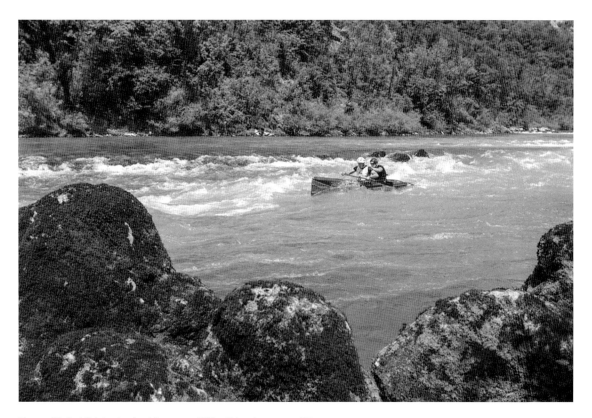

Figure 11.9 Athletes in double canoe (C2) wildwater competition.

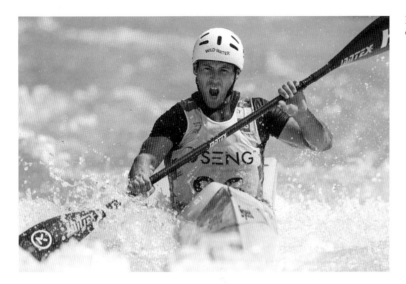

Figure 11.10 K1 wildwater competitor.

Dragon boat

Originating in ancient China, dragon boat paddling is becoming a global canoe discipline at both competitive and recreational levels. These long canoes are paddled by 20 paddlers or, in the smaller version, by 10 athletes using single-bladed paddles. Often, the dragon boat will be elaborately decorated, and include a drummer and steersperson or sweep.

Dragon boat paddling is an excellent entry to canoe racing. Participation results in predictable improvements in fitness, it is suitable for all ages, it rewards teamwork, and it is fun to paddle. There are large dragon boat festivals that are popular with recreational paddlers, clubs, and corporate teams. Other groups are using this activity as a medical intervention to restore health.

Timing and technique are critical indicators of performance; the paddle is small in volume, and success in this sport is based on synchrony paddling together. There are various race distances (200–2000 m in international competitions), and strength, muscular endurance, as well as aerobic capacity are essential. The competitor is sitting and paddles only on one side of the boat. Proper technique requires rotation through the pelvis

and sacroiliac, and lumbar spine strain can occur. Impingement syndrome of the top shoulder is a frequent problem (Figures 11.11 and 11.12).

Ocean racing

Ocean racing is the latest canoeing discipline to fall under ICF governance. This activity includes long-distance surf ski, sea kayak, and Va'a racing. *Va'a* means "boat" or "canoe" in Samoan, Tahitian, and Hawaiian, and it is recognized as meaning "outrigger canoe" throughout the world. To compete in ocean racing, athletes require both endurance fitness and boat skills. An extremely popular sport in warm coastal regions, ocean racing is huge in places such as Australia, California, Hawaii, and South Africa. Athletes in surf skis can expect to ride large wind-driven waves as well as the challenge of paddling in 20+ knot wind conditions. Limiting factors to performance are aerobic capacity, hydration, fuel, and avoidance of thermal and overuse injuries. Va'a is very popular, and races are conducted in single and six-person boats. There are sprint races as well as distances that can vary from approximately 10 km to multiday races over ultra-long distances (Figures 11.13–11.15).

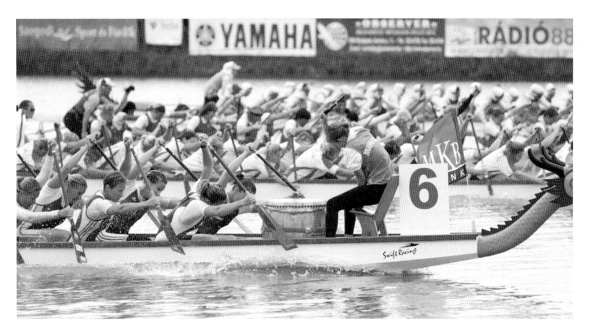

Figure 11.11 Dragon boat competition.

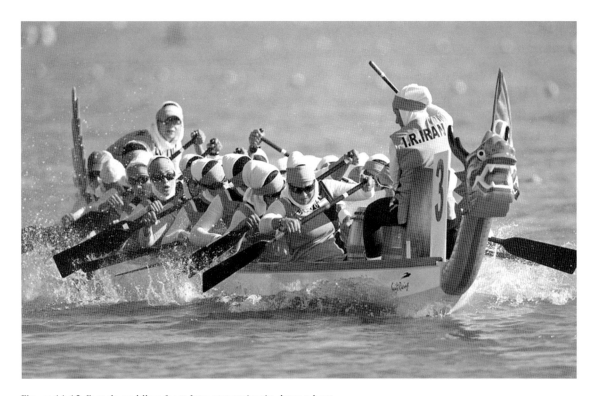

Figure 11.12 Female paddlers from Iran competing in dragon boat.

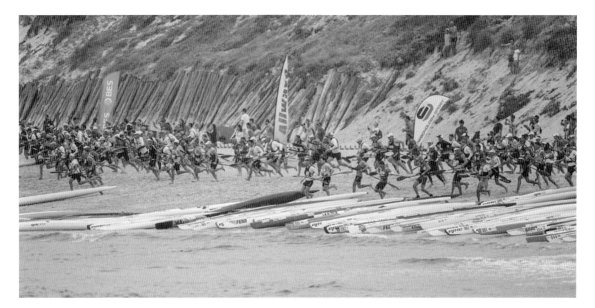

Figure 11.13 The start of a surf ski race.

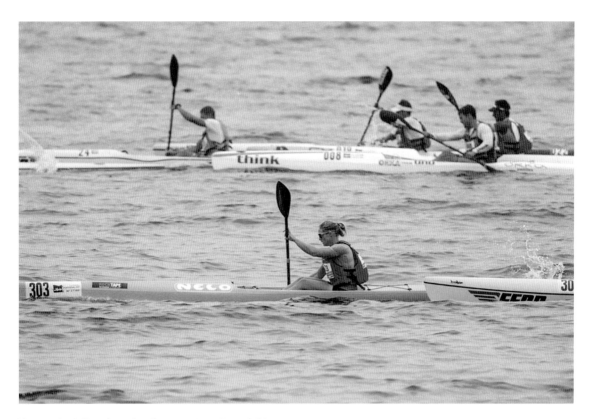

Figure 11.14 Female and male competitors in surf ski.

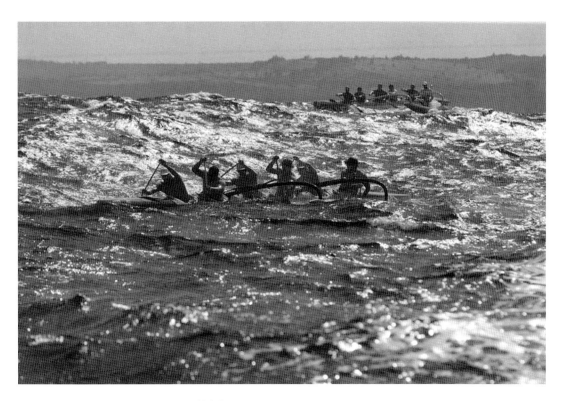

Figure 11.15 Six-person outrigger canoe (OC6) competitors in open-ocean racing.

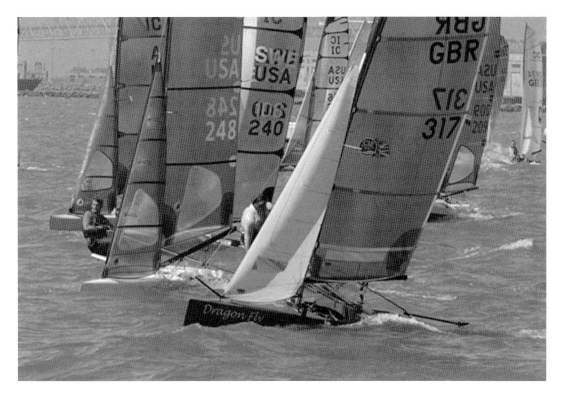

Figure 11.16 Canoe sailing.

Canoe sailing

Canoe sailing has a rich history in the ICF. It began as a sport in Europe in the nineteenth century, when canoes for competition and recreational purposes appeared. John MacGregor, the builder of the celebrated kayak *Rob Roy*, founded the British Royal Canoe Club in 1866, and before long the members of the Canoe Club were developing specialized craft for racing with a rudder and sail (Figures 11.16 and 11.17). These crafts have evolved, and the sport is now highly technical. Athletes sail small, sleek canoes that are propelled by large racing sails that harness the power of the wind. These are capable of high speed, creating some great racing. There are considerable physical demands, and muscular endurance, agility, and stamina are necessary to excel in competition. Upper-extremity tendinopathy, back strain, and shoulder strain are common problems.

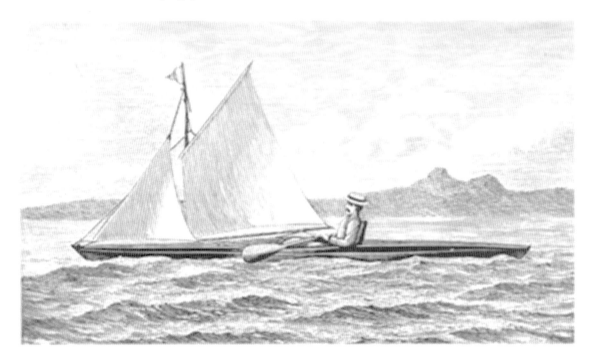

Figure 11.17 John MacGregor, founder of the British Royal Canoe Club, in the *Rob Roy*.

Index

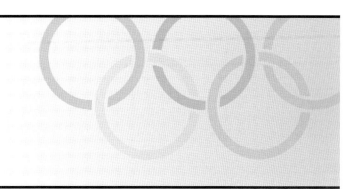

Canoeing, First Edition. Edited by Don McKenzie and Bo Berglund.
© 2019 International Olympic Committee. Published 2019 by John Wiley & Sons Ltd.